Vaibhav Dadu

The Vimana Sthana of the Charaka Samhita as a Knowledge and Measurement Unit

Anchor Academic
Publishing

Dadu, Vaibhav: The Vimana Sthana of the Charaka Samhita as a Knowledge and
Measurement Unit, Hamburg, Anchor Academic Publishing 2016

Buch-ISBN: 978-3-96067-086-5
PDF-eBook-ISBN: 978-3-96067-586-0
Druck/Herstellung: Anchor Academic Publishing, Hamburg, 2016

Bibliografische Information der Deutschen Nationalbibliothek:
Die Deutsche Nationalbibliothek verzeichnet diese Publikation in der Deutschen
Nationalbibliografie; detaillierte bibliografische Daten sind im Internet über
http://dnb.d-nb.de abrufbar.

Bibliographical Information of the German National Library:
The German National Library lists this publication in the German National Bibliography.
Detailed bibliographic data can be found at: http://dnb.d-nb.de

All rights reserved. This publication may not be reproduced, stored in a retrieval system
or transmitted, in any form or by any means, electronic, mechanical, photocopying,
recording or otherwise, without the prior permission of the publishers.

Das Werk einschließlich aller seiner Teile ist urheberrechtlich geschützt. Jede Verwertung
außerhalb der Grenzen des Urheberrechtsgesetzes ist ohne Zustimmung des Verlages
unzulässig und strafbar. Dies gilt insbesondere für Vervielfältigungen, Übersetzungen,
Mikroverfilmungen und die Einspeicherung und Bearbeitung in elektronischen Systemen.

Die Wiedergabe von Gebrauchsnamen, Handelsnamen, Warenbezeichnungen usw. in
diesem Werk berechtigt auch ohne besondere Kennzeichnung nicht zu der Annahme,
dass solche Namen im Sinne der Warenzeichen- und Markenschutz-Gesetzgebung als frei
zu betrachten wären und daher von jedermann benutzt werden dürften.

Die Informationen in diesem Werk wurden mit Sorgfalt erarbeitet. Dennoch können
Fehler nicht vollständig ausgeschlossen werden und die Diplomica Verlag GmbH, die
Autoren oder Übersetzer übernehmen keine juristische Verantwortung oder irgendeine
Haftung für evtl. verbliebene fehlerhafte Angaben und deren Folgen.

Alle Rechte vorbehalten

© Anchor Academic Publishing, Imprint der Diplomica Verlag GmbH
Hermannstal 119k, 22119 Hamburg
http://www.diplomica-verlag.de, Hamburg 2016
Printed in Germany

ACKNOWLEDGEMENTS

This gives me a great pleasure to acknowledge all those who have unswervingly promoted me to initiate and complete this intellectual task of authoring a book on my ideal Ayurveda classical of the Charaka Samhita especially the Vimana Sthana.

I heartly pay my sincere gratitude and obeisance to revered saint Shri Dadu Dayal Maharaja for bestowing his divine blessing that made me efficient enough to produce the work and the realization of the dream of authoring this book.

The gratitude towards my father late Shri Prakash Chandra Dadu and living legend my mother, Smt. Pushpa Devi cannot be expressed in words as they have been the foundation stone of my life. In their difficult times also, they continued to be a ray of sunshine for me.

No words of wisdom shall match my gratefulness towards my mentors and guides, my teachers especially Prof. Ram Babu Dwivedi, Prof. Mahesh Vyas and Dr. Hitesh Vyas for their invaluable supervision.

I acknowledge the teaching staff of Government Model Ayurveda College, Kolavada, Gandhinagar especially Dr. Rajesh Barvaliya, Dr. Naresh Jain, Dr. Swatiben Shah et al for their incredible support for this accomplishmemt.

I offer my sincere thanks to my family for their excellent understanding as the toil and dedication towards the completion of this text has taken a lot of time from their quota. I thank them for their support and assistance in every circumstance. Thank you all from my inner conscience.

Dr. Vaibhav Dadu

Preface

The *Charaka Samhita* is well known *Ayurveda* classic accredited for its deliberations on basic principles of *Ayurveda* that have remained the source of inspiration for the *Ayurveda* knowledge seekers. It is considered to be a complete text having no shortcomings. It is also termed as the *Kalpadruma* by the revered commentator *Gangadhara Roy*. As the legend says, the *Kalpadruma* is a tree that fulfils ones wish and has a plenty to offer. Similarly, the *Charaka Samhita* is a treasure trove of *Ayurveda* knowledge having unfathomable capacity to deliver the desired.

Although, all the eight sections of the text namely the *Sthaana* are unique in their content, the *Vimana Sthana* is a special unit conspicuous by its presence in the *Charaka Samhita*. The other classics like the *Sushruta Samhita* and the *Ashtanga Hridayam* of *Vagbhata* lack the *Vimana Sthana*. Therefore, the *Charaka Samhita* is a complete knowledge package for the *Ayurveda* seekers.

The *Vimana Sthana* is special as the definition of *Ayurveda* per se suggests the measurement of the beneficial and non-beneficial items for the life span as quoted in the *Charaka Samhita* -

> *Hitahitam sukham dukham ayustasyahitahitam*
> *Manam ca tatcha yatroktam Ayurvedah sa uchyate (Ch. Sa. Su.1)*

The *Vimana Sthana* is the knowledge and measurement unit. It specifies the mode of the measurement of the *doshadi* along with the very significant topic of the teaching & research methodology in *Ayurveda*. Therefore, here an attempt has been made to bring to light the significance of the *Vimana Sthana* in the expansion of the knowledge vistas of the ancient science of life, *Ayurveda* with special focus on the contemporary concept of the research and teaching methodology in *Ayurveda* system of medicine.

The author has made all the sincere efforts to achieve the goal of scientific elucidation of the facts based on the classical texts and commentaries along with his personal experience for which he may be credited. But in spite of all the efforts the lacunas may remain for which the author sincerely apologizes and seeks to rectify the same if brought to notice. The suggestions to improve are highly welcome as there is always a scope of improvement.

Thank you one and all

Yours,

(Dr. Vaibhav Dadu)

MD *Ayurveda* (Gold Medallist)

Index

S.No.	Name of the chapter	Page Number
01	*Charaka Samhita* – An Introduction	07 – 11
02	An Introduction to *Vimana Sthana*	12 – 15
03	*Vimana Sthana* and the basic principles of Ayurveda	16 – 34
04	*Vimana Sthana* – The *Pariksha sthana*	35 – 50
05	*Vimana Sthana* of *Charaka Samhita* – Applied aspect	51 – 64
06	Summary of the *Vimana Sthana* with its contemporary significance	65 – 72
07	References/Bibliography	73–74

Chapter 1

Charaka Samhita - An Introduction

The *Ayurveda* literature mainly the *Charaka Samhita* is a knowledge encyclopaedia considered as the best amongst the major triad or the *brihattrayee*. The other two are the *Sushruta Samhita* and the *Ashtanga Hridayam*. The formation of *Charaka Samhita* per se signifies the concept of literary research in *Ayurveda*.

The formation of the *Charaka Samhita* has been done in four stages:

a. **The narrator *Atreya*** – The available *Charaka Samhita* was narrated to the seer *Agnivesha* by the seer *Atreya*. Thus the *Guru Atreya* laid down the foundation of the greatest text of *Ayurveda* known as *Charaka Samhita*. His period is believed to be around 1000 B.C. i.e. 3000 years back.

b. **The primary author, *Agnivesha*** – The disciple of the teacher *Atreya* and *having* a sharp intellect accredited for the creation of the first text of the *Ayurveda* in a very concise form known as the *tantra*, the *Agnivesha*. Thus the narrator *Atreya* and the disciple *Agnivesha* share the same page in the history. The deliberations on the four limbs of treatment i.e. *Chikitsa Chatushpada* in the lines of the *Upanishads* and the concept of the wishes or desires is an indication of his might in the *Ayurveda* knowledge.

c. **The secondary author or the redactor, *Charaka*** (2nd Century B.C.) *Charaka* is one of the most well known names associated with *Ayurveda*. One of the stalwarts of *Ayurveda* who has redacted the *Agnivesha Tantra* and made it to the *Saṁhita* form known as *Charaka Saṁhita*. *Charaka* is considered to be an incarnation of the lord of the serpents, *Shesha*. Also, he is considered to be the community which was the branch of *Krishna Yajurveda*. He is also believed to be a nomadic sage. The contributions of *Charaka* include the description of the six categories, epistemology of the school of *Nyaya* and the inclusion of the disciplinary regimen known as *Swasthavritta* in *Ayurveda* parlance.

   d. Dridhbala (4th century) – The final strata of the completion of the *Charaka Samhita* is the addition of the chapters missing from the erstwhile text redacted by the seer *Charaka*. Thus, the missing 41 chapters (17 of the *Chikitsa Sthana,* 12 of the *Kalpa Sthana* and 12 of the *Siddhi Sthana).* The methodology used by the *Dridhbala* is the selective and the collective methodology called the *Unchha* and *Shila Vritti* respectively.

The classification of *Charaka Samhita*:

The *Charaka Samhita* is divided into eight sections or *Sthana* namely the *Sootra, Nidana, Vimana, Shareera, Indriya, Chikitsit, Kalpa & Siddhi Sthana* respectively. The sequence of these sections is of great significance as it is in tandem with the aims and objectives of the indigenous system of medicine, *Ayurveda*. The first and foremost target is the maintenance of health by following the *Ayurveda* system of life. The methodology of *Ayurveda* living and the Basic doctrine of *Ayurveda* which is its foundation are vividly explained in the first section or the *Sootra Sthana* known as the 'brain' of the *Charaka Samhita* . The essence of the knowledge of the whole text is extracted in its *Sootra Sthana*. The whole treatise is directed by the *Sootra Sthana*. The predominance of the *Sootra Sthana* can be gauged by its analogy to the nectar. The *Sootra Sthana* is the nectar of knowledge and is the collection of all the basics of *Ayurveda* medicine. All the three major treatises namely the *Charaka Samhita, Sushruta Samhita* and the *Ashtanga Hridayam* accord the highest importance to this first section called as the *Sootra Sthana*. The *Charaka Samhita sootra Sthana* is unique as it has been divided into quartets which is a group of four chapters, thus the total of thirty chapters are categorized under the seven groups of four chapters known as *Sapta Chatushka* (28 chapters) and the remaining two are the collection of the information termed as the *Sangraha dwaya*. These quartets convey all the basic information of the *Ayurveda* system of medicine but the information is in coded form which needs to be deciphered in all its merit. This paper therefore presents an in depth analysis of the quartet methodology of the *Charaka Samhita* with special reference to the fundamentals of the science of life, *Ayurveda*.

The *Nidana Sthana* has eight chapters which detail the points of diagnosis of a disease. The eight chapters are in line of the eight tissues. The *Jwara* is the disease of the *Rasa*, the *Raktapitta* is the disease of the *Rakta*, *Gulma* is the disease of the *Mamsa*, *Prameha* afflicts the *Meda* and so on. The fundamentals of the diagnosis mentioned in this section are used in the *Ayurvedic* understanding of the diseases hitherto unknown.

The *Vimana Sthana* is a special section of *Charaka Samhita* as it is conspicuous by its absence in all other treatises of *Ayurveda*. The detailed analysis of the *Vimana Sthana* is described in the coming chapters.

The *Sharira Sthana* follows the *Vimana Sthana*. This section as the name suggests promulgates on the various aspects of the birth and formation and development of the body. The eight chapters of the *Sharira Sthana* also known as the *Ashraya Sthana* deal with the detailed view of the embryology, parturition, neonatal care along with the unique philosophical description of the body made up of twenty – four elements, the mind and the anatomical entities like the bones, organs-sub organs, blood vessels *et al.*

Then the next is the *Indriya or Arishta Sthana* i.e. the section dealing with the prognostic signs and symptoms. The twelve chapters describe the signs of imminent death known as *Arishta*. These signs include the signs of the five objects of the senses, the dreams *et al.* This section needs a lot of research to be conducted as it has the potential of a possible solution to the ever increasing menace of the untreatable disease conditions and manifestations.

After the ascertainment of the disease condition, the physician starts the treatment procedure. The mode of treatment is explained in the section called *Aushadha Sthana* or the *Chikitsa Sthana*. There is unanimity on the supremacy of the *Chikitsa Sthana* of the *Charaka Samhita*. The thirty chapters *Aushadha Sthana* start with the lucid in-depth description of the *Rasayana and Vajikarana* therapies. The *Rasayana* is analogous to the modern day geriatrics and anti-oxidant therapies while the *Vajikarana* postulates the remedy to the sexual disorders particularly the cases of infertility or impotency. After these two chapters, the vivid description of the disease with its line of treatment mainly the treatment principle has been described. The diseases ranging from the *jwara* to the twenty conditions related to the Gynaecology have been explained with their unique treatment plan.

After the deliberations on the mode and principle of *Ayurveda* treatment, the next section of eight chapters of the *kalpa or Vikalpa Sthana* deals with the choice and preparation of the medicine in various combinations. These combinations are mainly associated with the medicines of the purification therapy or the *Panchkarma*.

The last section is the *Siddhi Sthana* of twelve chapters. *Siddhi* means the successful accomplishment. Thus, the *Siddhi Sthana* deals with the process and management of the untoward reactions or the complications as may arise due to the faulty prescription or procedure of the *Panchkarma*. In the last chapter the exposition of the cannons of exposition i.e. *tantrayuktis* has been elaborated.

Thus from the above deliberation it is clear that the *Charaka Samhita* is the foremost classic of *Ayurveda* acting as the beacon of light for the *Ayurveda* academicians and practitioners. It is generally accepted that the more we read and understand *Charaka Samhita*, the novelty in expansion of the knowledge vistas is certain. The *Charaka Samhita* is the *Ayurveda* encyclopaedia as it has the answers to the most of the health related problems of the society. The harmony with the nature is the crux of discussion in the *Charaka Samhita*. The unanimity between the man and the environment is the cause of successful *Ayurveda* therapy. The 120 chapters of *Charaka Samhita* have a definite science hidden in them which needs to be understood minutely in the present day scientific light. The *Charaka Samhita* has an unfathomable capacity to answer the contemporary intriguing medical questions.

Here an attempt has been made to understand one section namely the *Vimana Sthana* of the *Charaka Samhita* in the scientific light. The *Vimana Sthana* is unique section that has been taken as the knowledge and measurement unit.

Chapter 2

An Introduction to *Vimana Sthana*

As stated, the *Vimana Sthana* is a unique and detailed section having an explanation contributed by *Charaka* as no other seer amongst the highly regarded three major classics of *Ayurveda* describes the *Vimana Sthana* as a separate section. Although the *Bhela* and *kashyapa Samhita* have a *Vimana Sthana* but this section is either controversial or deficient. This section bears great significance as the definition of *Ayurveda* per se includes the concept of the measurement called as *mana* in *Ayurveda* parlance. The position of the *Vimana Sthana* also bears significance as all the sections and chapters in *Charaka Samhita* have a specific sequence in tandem with their utility in the treatment or method of maintaining the health. The *Vimana Sthana* has been positioned between the *Nidana Sthana* and the *Sharira Sthana*. The position after the *Nidana Sthana* is valid as it is the confirmation of the need of the measurement of the *doshadi* i.e. *dosha, desha, kala, bheshaja, sharira, sara, ahara, sattva, satmya prakriti et.al.* after the ascertainment of the diagnosis described in the *Nidana Sthana*. The *Vimana Sthana* therefore is the specific section dedicated to the measurement or the knowledge unit. The measurement of the beneficial and non-beneficial is the base of *Ayurveda* methodology of health maintenance and treatment of the disease. It is essential to have a proper knowledge of the measurement as the later is the base of the standardization. The process of the standardization of the *Ayurveda* components of the *dosha et al* is necessary to pursue the research activity in *Ayurveda*. The research is the facts supported with figures that involve the measurement which is the crux of discussion in the *Vimana Sthana*. In fact, the eighth chapter of the *Vimana Sthana* is the treasure of the Basic Principles of research in *Ayurveda*. Thus, the *Vimana Sthana* of the *Charaka Samhita* is the foundation stone or the guiding principle for the pursuance of the research activity in the contemporary progressive but classical science of the Indian medicine, *Ayurveda*.

The chapters of the *Vimana Sthana* and their *abhidheya* i.e. the topic of discussion as knowledge units:

There are eight chapters of the *Vimana Sthana* of *Charaka Samhita*. The details of them is tabulated below.

Name of the Chapter	Topic of discussion/Knowledge units
Rasa Vimana	- *Rasa, dravya, dosha vikara prabhava* - The knowledge of the effect of the *doshadi-* expected as well as unexpected. - Concept of the *Vikritivishamasamaveta & prakritisamasamaveta* - Conditional use of the three common medicines namely the *pippali. Kshara & lavana.* - Basic factors of dietetics or the *ahara vidhi visheshayatana.*
Trividhakukshiya Vimana	- Application of the dietetic factors. - Volume and quantity of food with its beneficial and non-beneficial effects. - Unripe food/*Ama* with its diagnosis, types and treatment principle. - Causative factor of disease with its measurement.

Janapadodhwamsaniya Vimana	- Epidemiology in *Ayurveda* - Common factors of disease - Man and environment (Ecological Considerations) - Non-judicial use of the resources by the human being - Compared with the contemporary menace of the pollution/climate change
Trividharogavishesha Vijnaniya Vimana	- Special knowledge of the diagnostic units - Application of the epistemology of philosophy mainly the *Nyaya*. - Triad of the 'Knowledge units' (*trividha jnana samgraha*)
Sroto Vimana	- Vivid description of the pathways/chammels termed as *Srotasa*. - *Srotasa* as the inevitable factors of disease.
Roganika Vimana	- Knowledge of the disease groups with their classification - Diagnostic factors of the main and supporting causative factor of the *dosha*. - Diagnostic characters of the *agni, dosha* with their treatment principles.
Vyadhitarupiya Vimana	- Specific knowledge of the diseased w.s.r to their mental strength. - *Krimi Vijnana* i.e. knowledge of the various parasites/germs with their control.
Rogabhishagjitiya Vimana	- Knowledge and its examination. - The clear knowledge of the medicine.

	- The methods of the examination/*pariksha*. - Ten fold examination of the patient with its measurement as *pravara* (high), *madhya* (medium) and *avara* (low). - Basics of research activity in *Ayurveda*. - Importance and necessity of the examination/ research activity. - Classification of the drugs.

From the above table it becomes clear that the *Vimana Sthana* serves as a treasure trove as it postulates the knowledge and the measurement units in the *Ayurveda* system of medicine. A plethora of topics needed to be known by an aspiring *Ayurveda* practitioner and the academician have been dealt with in detail in this section which makes the *Charaka Samhita* as the complete text of the *Ayurveda* system of medicine amongst all the available texts.

The measurement units of the weight, capacity (volume), length and time have been explained and utilized to their potential in the *Ayurveda* system of treatment of the disease. Thus, the *mana* i.e. measurement which is the most significant factor of *Ayurveda* is vividly explained in the *Vimana Sthana* of the *Charaka Samhita*. The knowledge of the measurement units have their application in every aspect of the *Ayurveda* thinking which will be described in the systematic study of various chapters ahead.

Chapter 3

Vimana Sthana and the basic principles of *Ayurveda*

Vimana Sthana is the treasure trove of the basic principles of *Ayurveda*. The strong foundation of the *Ayurveda* system of medicine is based upon the concept of the measurement described in the *Vimana Sthana*. The two aims of *Ayurveda* i.e. the maintenance of health and the treatment of the disease are achieved by following the *Ayurveda* lifestyle and the *Ayurveda* principles of treatment. The *Vimana Sthana* is the knowledge unit and thus it becomes mandatory to understand the various basic principles of *Ayurveda* promulgated in the *Vimana Sthana* having application in the achievement of the goal of healthy long life.

The definition of *siddhanta* (principle in modern parlance) has been postulated in the *Vimana Sthana* of the *Charaka Samhita*. The principle known as *Siddhaanta* in *Ayurveda* signifies all that which is valid and true. The theory that is demonstrated to be true & valid after repeated examination by a number of examiners is termed as *Siddhanta/Principle*. The *Nyaya* philosophy also defines *Siddhanta* as the subject accepted after being validated through various evidences. Thus the *Vimana Sthana* of the *Charaka Samhita* is full of the Basic Principles of *Ayurveda* sans which the two aims of the eternal science of *Ayurveda* cannot be achieved.

The *Ayurveda* treatises and Philosophy both accept the four types of *Siddhānta*. They are:

(a) The ***Sarvatantra Siddhanta*** **(Widely approved principle)** - The *Siddhanta* approved by all the treatises is the *Sarvatantra Siddhanta* like the presence of *Nidana* and *Vyadhi*.

Thus, the concepts of *Panchamahabhoota Siddhanta, Roga-Rogi Pariksha Siddhanta, Ayu Siddhanta, Dosha- Dhatu- Mala Siddhanta, Agni Siddhanta et al* is the *Sarvatantra Siddhanta*.

(b) The *Pratitantra Siddhanta* (Approved by a particular clan) -

The *Siddhanta* approved by a particular treatise/s but not widely agreed upon is the *Pratitantra Siddhanta* like the approval of eight *rasa* by the others while six *rasa* here. There is a difference of opinion between different authors.

The suggestions of the enumeration of *Agni* differ from one *Acharya*/Treatise to the other as is the case with the theories regarding the first organ to develop in the foetus.

These *Siddhanta* which differ from treatise to treatise are the *Pratitantra Siddhanta*.

(c) The *Adhikarana Siddhanta* (Principle of reference) -

The topic/subject discussed under one *Siddhanta* implies the other unstated topic/subject is categorized under the umbrella of *Adhikarana Siddhanta* like the statement suggesting the inaction of the liberated soul suggests that there is existence of the actions, their results and rebirths.

Like the *sootra* pertaining to the conditions of curability (*sadhyata*) of a disease as the *dushya* and *prakriti* should not be the causative *dosha*. This *sootra* albeit clearly mentions the conditions of curability of the disease, also implies that there is existence of disease which has certain conditions of curability-incurability based on the entities of body viz *dosha, dushya, prakriti* et al. These *Siddhanta* having implied/inferred valid topics/subjects is termed as the *Adhikarana Siddhanta*.

(d) The *Abhyupagama Siddhanta* (Accepted theory to be validated) -

The *Abhyupagama Siddhanta* is the theory which is not validated, explicated and tested but accepted during a course of discussion like the narration of supremacy of *dravya,* supremacy of *Guna* etc.

Therefore, it contradicts the definition of *Siddhanta* and shouldn't be classified as *Siddhanta*. But, instead it is rightly placed as *Siddhanta* because it paves the way for the formation of *Siddhanta*. The 'untested theory/hypothesis' put forth is tested and examined and if found true, becomes a *Siddhanta*. All the various opinions/questions of *Aacharyas* regarding a particular matter of debate are termed as the *Abhyupagama Siddhanta*.

Principles of *Ayurveda* dietetics – These principles include the deliberations on the factors determining the beneficial or non-beneficial effects of the food. The principles of dietetics include the concept of *prakriti* (nature of the food), *karana* (transformation including the food processing), *samyoga* (combination of food items), *rashi* (quantity of the food), *desha* (place of origin, development, processing and consumption of the food), *kala* (time of food intake), *upayogasamstha* (code of the food intake) *and upayokta* (consumer). These eight factors are termed as the *ashta aharavidhi visheshayatana.*

Along with these eight factors, the whole concept of the proper methodology of food intake like the consumption of the fresh food explained in the terms of *ushna* (hot), unctuous, *et al* are very significant in dietetics in *Ayurveda* science. The food is said to be the life (*prana*) in *Ayurveda*. The food is responsible for development and maintenance of the body. Some of the seers like *Kashyapa* call food as the *Mahabhaishajya* (great medicine).

Principles of diagnosis – The *Vimana Sthana* of the *Charaka Samhita* ponders over all the aspects of *Ayurveda* diagnosis and treatment. The chapter five of the *Vimana Sthana* namely the *Srotovimana adhyaya* is a guide to all the diagnostic principles as the *Ayurveda* system of medicine ascribes the progression of disease to the vitiation of the *srotasa* or the channels. This chapter presents an in-depth analysis of the various definitions of the *srotasa* and their role in the nutrition of the body as well as in the disease production. The causative factors of the vitiation of the *srotasa* and their manifestations are explained in this chapter.

Similarly, the concept of the *Agni* as the cause of disease when vitiated is also taken care of in the *Vimana Sthana*. The chapter six namely the *Roganeeka Vimana* postulates the four types of the factor of transformation i.e. *agni* as *teekshna* (strong), *manda* (weak), *sama* (even) and *vishama* (uneven). Apart from the *sama* which is the desired, the rest three represent a predominance of one or the other *dosha* (the unit when vitiated is the potent and independent cause of the disease). *Ayurveda* believes in the involvement of the *agni* as one of the causative factors of the disease. Agni is indeed the factor of transformation and thus its normalcy leads to a proper transformation i.e. production of the desired and its transformation thereafter. Also, the *Vimana Sthana* mentions diagnostic importance of the *doshas*. When there is an involvement of the two or three *doshas* in a disease, the *dosha* which is independent, manifests itself and is vitiated and pacified as per the classical view is said to be the chief or the *anubandhya* while the other *dosha/doshas* which are dependent, manifests in later stage and do not follow the classical line of treatment is the *anubandha* or the supportive. This principle of diagnosis is important in the nomenclature of the hitherto unknown diseases as the disease should be named according to the major causative *dosha*.

The *Vimana Sthana* mentions three categories of people who are usually prone to diseases i.e. they are generally suffering from ailments. Based on the predominance of the *dosha,* they are termed as the *Vatika* (predominance of *Vata* and therefore easily prone to the *Vatika* disorders), *Paittika* (predominance of *Pitta* and therefore easily prone to the *Paittika* disorders) and the *Shleshmalah* (predominance of *Kapha* and therefore easily prone to the *Kaphaja* disorders).

The chapter seven of the *Vimana Sthana* namely the *Vyaadhitarupiya Vimana* is a further advancement of knowledge of the diagnosis as a mere appearance may lead to faulty diagnosis. The chapter describes the two types of patients as the first category is strong mentally and physically and can bear the pain. These patients although suffering from a serious disease present their case as the disease is trivial while the other category is the patients having a weak mental built and therefore cannot bear slightest of pain. Such people make a trivial complaint appear as the serious disease. These two categories are known as *guruvyadhita* and *laghuvyadhita* respectively. This is significant in diagnosis as the faulty diagnosis will definitely lead to the faulty treatment which may aggravate the disease or suffering.

Likewise the *Vyadhitarupiya Vimana* also presents a new aspect of disease into limelight which is the concept of worms/germs termed as *krimi* in *Ayurveda*. Some scholars even compare this deliberation to the modern concept of microorganisms and the parasites. This chapter of the *Vimana Sthana* describes the types of *krimi* along with their characters and line of treatment.

Moreover, the clinical methods of diagnosis of a disease is also enunciated in the *Vimana Sthana* as it presents the following examinations of the disease and the patient:

a. The *trividha roga vijnaneeya adhyaya* (chapter on the three specific parameters of the examination of the disease) presents the applied aspect of the epistemology of the Indian Philosophy. The three tools of examination of a disease are the *pratyaksha* (direct observation), *anumana* (inference) and the *aptopadesha/shabda* (authoritative testimony). These three major tools of examination find their utility in the diagnosis in every science of medicine. The direct observation deals with the direct observation possible through the five sense organs. The methods of physical examination involve the inspection, palpation, auscultation and interrogation, all unthinkable sans the senses. The inference or the *anumana* is the logical reasoning based upon the established relationship of the cause and effect. The authoritative testimony or the *shabda/aptopadesha* is the established and trustworthy word which is approved and accepted by all. The renowned texts like the *Ayurveda* classics and the religious scriptures are accepted in their might.

b. The *dasha vidha rogi pareeksha* (tenfold examination of the diseased) – The tenfold examination of the diseased is the crux of the chapter eight of the *Vimana Sthana* of *Charaka Samhita* namely the *Rogabhishagjitiya Vimana*. This tenfold examination is done to assess the status of strength of the *dosha* and life span. It includes the examination of :

  i. *Prakriti* (Inherent nature) – The concept of the *prakriti* or the innate character or predisposition is a unique concept of the *Ayurveda* philosophy. The *Vimana Sthana* chapter eight presents an in-depth evaluation of the *prakriti* based on the qualities of the constituent *dosha*. Although the concept of *prakriti* is available in the *sutra Sthana*, the first section of the *Charaka Samhita* itself but its detailed knowledge and evaluation is available in the *Vimana*

Sthana. The characters of a *prakriti* are manifested in the body in tandem with the quality of the constituting *dosha*. This is measured in the case of the composite (due to two or three *dosha*) *prakriti* as well. This concept is of great clinical importance as the curability of the disease depends on the relation of the *prakriti* i.e. natural predisposition with the aggravated causative factor of the disease i.e. the *dosha*.

ii. *Vikriti* (Pathology) – The *Vikriti* means the pathology. The points to examine the pathology are six viz. cause (*hetu*), potent factor of disease (*dosha*), secondary factors or substratum of a disease (*dushya*), natural character (*prakriti*), habitat (*desha*) and the unavoidable factor of the time (*kala*). The strength of these six factors decides the status of the pathology. A disease or pathological state is said to be strong if the strength of the six factors is equally powerful.

iii. *Saara* (Status of the tissue) – The tissue known as *dhatu* in *Ayurveda* parlance is the abode of *dosha*. The vitiated *dosha* afflict the *dhatus* (tissues) to produce a disease. Status of the might of a *dhatu* is assessed in the form of *saara* i.e. the status of its quality. The *saara* is assessed in three varieties i.e. the best, medium and low categories. The best category of *saarata* is desirable as it represents a strong body. The eight varieties of *saara* have been described in the *Vimana Sthana*. Again there is a need of standardization of these characteristics which will be a great achievement for the medical sciences. Along with the status of a *dhatu*, the *saarata* also conveys the quality of life a person is expected to live. Ex. the best quality of reproductive tissue known as *shukra* bestows power, happiness, respectability and fulfilment of the physical desires of a person.

iv. *Samhanana* (Physical Compactness) – The physical compactness involves a proper distribution of muscular and bony tissue. A person is physically strong i.e. able to bear pain when he/she is having an optimum distribution of muscles at their required sites.

v. *Pramana* (Size/Measurement of the body parts/components) – This examination validates the *Vimana Sthana* as the measurement unit. The optimum size of the major components of body has been listed here. However, the unit of measurement is the persons own finger i.e. the *anguli pramana.* This again requires to be standardized through a sincere research activity. The optimum length of a person is said to be 84 *anguli.* This optimum length ensures better strength of the body.

vi. *Sattva* (Status of the mental strength) –The *Ayurveda* is probably the first ever medical science to incorporate the mind as an integral part of the body. The site of health and disease is the physical body and the mind alike. The mental status affects the physique and vice versa. The mind is categorized into three varieties according to the strength. The *pravara* (higher grade) *sattva* is that which bestows the self confidence and capability to withstand the adversaries at one's own while the *madhyama* (medium grade) *sattva* is characterized by the reliance on others for ones strength i.e. these persons face the challenges/adversaries depending on the others' advice. The *hina* (lower grade) *sattva* is undesirable as this makes a person lose his/her confidence which is very difficult to regain even after the words of wisdom from the well wishers. This gradation is again very significant in the contemporary era as the mental disorders are on a rise and people taking the extreme steps of even committing suicide or becoming drug addicts.

vii. *Satmya* (Suitability/adaptability) – The concept of *satmya* envisages the adaptability of the body on prolonged exposure. The concept of staple food expects the *satmya*. The person desiring for a good health should have an exposure of all the six *rasa* (tastes) of food. This can be compared to the concept of balanced diet in the contemporary sciences.

viii. *Aharashakti* (Capacity of intake and digestion of the food) – The food is the cause of life of the living things. The quantity of food depends upon the ingestion and digestion power. The factor for the digestion i.e. the *agni* is the cause of all the diseases as it is the faulty transformation that leads to the abnormal production of *dhatus/tissues*. Thus, *aharashakti* (power of ingestion and digestion) is an important parameter of the examination of a patient and diagnosis.

ix. *Vyayama Shakti* (Physical ability) – The *vyayama shakti* is a test of physical ability. The contemporary treadmill test for the heart function and the spirometrical tests for the lung capacity are an excellent modernization of the test of physical strength and thus the *vyayama shakti*. In the diseases of the respiratory system and the cardiac system, the best diagnosis is through the *vyayama shakti*. This examination is through the inference as the direct observation of the same is not possible. The capability to endure more physical strain indicates better *vyayama shakti*.

x. *Vayah* (Assessment of the age/lifespan) - The *Ayurveda* system of medicine presents the assessment of the age or *vayah*. The assessment of age is based upon the development of tissue and attainment of the *bala* or strength. The noteworthy feature of this examination is that there is a dominance of the *kapha* in the childhood, *pitta* in the youth and the *vata* in the old age.

Thus the *Vimana Sthana* of *Charaka Samhita* is a multispeciality knowledge and measurement unit providing myriad opportunities of the research activity in *Ayurveda*.

Also, the chapter 3 of the *Vimana Sthana* of *Charaka Samhita* namely the *Janapadodhvamsaniya adhyaya* presents an *Ayurvedic* view of the epidemiology. The common causative factors of an epidemic are the air, water, place/region/habitat and the time/season called as *vaayu, jala, desha & kala* in *Ayurveda* classics. The signs of the vitiation of the air, water and land are analogous with their pollution. However, the *kala* or the time as a cause of epidemic indicates the inappropriate season i.e. the deviation in the seasonal characters. Also there is a deliberation on the Hindu theory of the origin of the disease. All the diseases are said to be produced by the intellectual blasphemy known as the *prajnaparadha* having roots in the non-virtuous life or the *adharma*.

This concept may be understood in the scientific light as the human desires are beyond control and the greed for physical pleasure (both fall under the concept of intellectual blasphemy, *prajnaparadha*) is leading to the excess exploitation of the nature causing the climate change manifested in various natural disasters and diseases.

Principles of treatment:

The *Vimana Sthana* describes various principles of *Ayurveda* treatment like the treatment principle of improper transformed food. The treatment of the *amadosha* produced due to the improper digestion of the food is described in the chapter 2 namely the *trividhakuksheeya Vimana*. The treatment of the *alasaka* is described as the emesis and emaciation (fasting) therapy. The treatment principle of *visuchika* is the *lamghana* (emaciation) followed by the therapy used after the *virechana* (purgation). The sequence of the treatment should follow the condition of the factor for the digestion which is the *agni*. This includes the intake of the gruels made up of rice and varying amounts of water. This is an important method of the attainment of the normal health, the natural way. This chapter also describes the treatment modality of the *apatarpana* (emaciation/fasting). After the treatment based on the cause i.e. against the causative factor (*hetuviparita*) and if the desired result is not obtained, the disease specific treatment is to be used known as the *vyadhiviparita*. After the treatment i.e. the amelioration of the disease, the process to increase the strength is advised through the oil enema (*anuvasana vasti*) and the massage.

The treatment modality of *ama dosha* i.e. untransformed/undigested food has been explained in a sequence such that there are no untoward effects on the body and the strength is restored.

'Prevention is better than cure', this is a word of caution approved by the *Charaka Samhita* and the *Vimana Sthana*. To prevent an epidemic, it is important to maintain the harmony between man and the environment. By leading a virtuous life i.e. not misusing or judicially using of the natural resources along with the oath not to pollute the environment are the key factors of prevention of an epidemic. Also, the use of anti-oxidants or the *rasayana* is advised to check the menace of an epidemic.

As a measurement unit, the *Vimana Sthana* of *Charaka Samhita* again presents three measurements of the *apatarpana* (emaciation) therapy.

a. *Lamghana* (Therapy producing lightness) – This therapy is the first line of treatment. Although the details of the same have been narrated in the *Sutra Sthana* of *Charaka Samhita*, the measurement of the same hasn't been postulated. In the *Vimana Sthana* chapter three namely the *Janapadodhvamsaniya adhyaya* the measurement of the therapy of *lamghana* has been detailed as it is used when the strength of the *dosha* is weak. Through this therapy, the *vata* and *agni* increase to pacify the *dosha* just as the case with the little water which gets dried up with the air and heat.

b. *Lamghana-pachana* (Combination of the fasting/lightness therapy with the digestion) – When the strength of the *dosha* is more i.e. it cannot be controlled through the *lamghana*, this combined therapy of the *langha & pachana* is used. Just as the drying of water through the air, heat and addition of the soil or sand.

c. *Doshavasechana* (Expulsion of the *dosha*) – This strongest therapy is to be used in the cases of *doshas* of high strength. This involves the use of purgation therapy i.e. forceful expulsion of the vitiated *dosha*. This cures the disease as the forceful expulsion of water in the cases of deluge or water logging.

Therefore, the *langhana* is to be used when the strength of the *dosha* and the diseased is less, the *langhana - pachana* is advised when the strength is medium while the extreme *doshavasechana* is the treatment of choice when the strength of the *dosha* and the diseased is optimum.

Similarly in the chapter five, *Srotovimana adhyaya,* the principle of the treatment of the diseases of some of the *srotasa* has been narrated. The treatment of the vitiated *mutravaha srotasa* is that of the *mutrakricchra* (dysurea), the treatment of the vitiated *purishavaha srotasa* is that of the *atisara* (diarrhoea) while the treatment of the *swedavaha srotasa* is that of the *jwara* (fever). In the vitiation of the *pranavaha, udakavaha* and the *annavaha srotasa* the advised treatment is that of the *shwasa* (dysnoea/asthma), *trisna upashamani* (pacifying the thirst) and the *amapradosha* (non – transformed state) respectively.

In the chapter 6, *roganika Vimana,* the Basic Principles of treatment of the most potent factor of the disease, *dosha* have been described. These principles of treatment find their application in the care of the diseases not hitherto described in the classical texts of *Ayurveda*.

Chapter 7 of the *Vimana Sthana* namely the *Vyadhita rupiya Vimana* introduces a new concept of *krimi* along with its treatment procedure. The three principles of the control of the parasites in the body (*krimi*) are the *apakarshana* (pulling out/expulsion), *prakritivighaat* (use of the ant parasite diet and medicine) and the *nidana parivarjana* (renunciation of the cause).

Principles of research:

In the *Rogabhishagjitiya Vimana,* there is a detailed description of the *pariksha* or examination. The ten points of examination are termed as the *dashavidha parikshya bhava*. These ten points of examination are the base of every research activity. These ten points of examinations are:

- *Kaarana* (The Research Scholar) – This is the scholar who pursues a Research project. The Research scholar along with the knowledge of the concerned subject should essentially possess the qualities of perseverance and effort.
- The *karana* (The tools/instruments) – These are the tools or the instruments that are used by the research scholar in his due course of scientific experimentation and reasoning. This includes all the materials used during the research procedure.
- The *kaarya Yoni* (The source of the problem) - The material or the essential cause of the problem which has transformed into a subject of Research/Investigation. This involves the search of the source of the problem as the source gives the clue to the approach towards the solution of the problem.
- The *kaarya* (The manifestation/ transformation desired) – The aim and objective which are to be achieved by the research scholar. It involves the solution to the problem for which the research activity has been undertaken.
- The *Kaarya phala* (The immediate result)- The immediate result and effect produced by the Research activity.
- The *Anubandha* (The contribution/ long time accomplishments) - The contribution that is bound to be associated with the research scholar in the positive or negative ways.
- The *Desha* (The Research Site/Place) – This concern with the area or the site of Research undertaken considering its pros and cons.
- The *Kaala* (Time/Duration of Research) – The time is an unavoidable factor in all the activities undertaken. The stipulated period of Research with its relation to the time is the importance of *kaala*.

- The *Pravritti* (Initiation/Effort) - The research scholar has to have the will or the desire to undertake the initiation or effort for his research project.
- The *Upaaya* (Method/Plan) – The best research plan that brings about the excellence in the scholar and utilization of the tools or the means. This involves the optimum utilization of the funds and the resources.

These above mentioned ten essentials for the pursuance of any research work decide the result or due course of action for the rectification of any shortcomings.

Similarly this chapter of the *Vimana Sthana* suggests the points of investigation of a drug which is applied in the research of a new drug or the existing drug. These points of drug research in *Ayurveda* are:

1. Nature (*Prakriti*) of the drug – Based on the constitution of the *panchamahabhuta* the nature of the drug is formed. Some may be hot while the others may be cold in potency.
2. Quality (*Guna*) of the drug i.e. the cause of its selection or rejection.
3. Special effect (*Prabhava*) of the drug – The concept of *prabhava* has been explained in the first chapter of the *Vimana Sthana* itself under the heading of the *vikriti vishama samaveta*. Some drugs act as per their qualities while others deviate or demonstrate some special effect due to the heterogeneous combination of the five basic elements, *panchamahabhuta*. Although there has to be a cause accountable for the special effect, the same needs to be searched.
4. Place of origin and growth (*Asmin deshe jatam*) – The *Charaka Samhita* and the *Vimana Sthana* explains vividly the harmony of the macrocosm (universe) with the macrocosm (man). The *desha* or a region (habitat) influences the nature and action of a drug. Based on the climatic and soil

condition, the drug and its action vary. The drugs from the Himalayas are cool in potency while the drugs hailing from the desert are hot in potency. Even the same species of a drug differs in quality or action according to the habitat.

5. Time and mode of collection (*Asmin ritau evam grihitam*) – The *kala* or the time is an unavoidable factor in *Ayurveda*. The time is the factor of production and destruction. The different parts of a plant are collected in special seasons based on their potencies.

6. Mode of storage and preservation *(Nihitam)* – To ensure throughout the year availability and the best maintenance of the potency (which is supposed to decrease continuously) it is very important to take care of the method of storage and preservation. The Good storage ensures the long life of a drug and is economically feasible.

7. Transformation or processing *(Upaskrutam)* – The raw drug needs a proper transformation to be converted into a usable form with an increased potency. This process is termed as *sanskara* in *Ayurveda* parlance. The GMP (Good manufacturing practice) is the key to the efficacy of a medication.

8. Dosage of the drug (*Anaya ca matraya yuktam*) – The dose of the drug depends on the condition of the disease and the status of the patient. The dosage also depends on the type of action of the drug whether the purification (*shodhana*) or pacification (*shamana*). A proper and desired dose of a poison can save one's life (as a drug) while even an elixir when consumed in an inappropriate dose can take away the life (as a poison).

Similarly the concept of *prakriti, agni et al* described in the *Vimana Sthana* are the points of research in *Ayurveda* in various specialities.

Moreover the fivefold statement or the *panchavayava vakya* described in the *Vimana Sthana* is also representative of the research methodology adopted in the contemporary research methodology as well. These five statements or points of research activity are:

a. *Pratijna* (Hypothesis) – The statement of the hypothesis to be validated or proved is the first step of research activity termed as *pratijna* by *Charaka*.

b. *Hetu* (Cause/source of Validation) – The sources (materials and methods) integral for the research activity. In *Ayurveda* system, it is the tools of examination described under the heading of *pramana* termed as *hetu*. After the formulation of a hypothesis it is essential to have the source of data and its validation thereafter. This collection of data and experimental design is placed under the materials and methods. *Ayurveda* accepts the supremacy of the four tools of examination basically explained in the Indian Philosophical school of *Nyaya*. These include the *pratyaksha* (direct observation), *anumana* (inference), *aptopadesha/shabda* (authoritative testimony) and the *upamana* (analogy). These four tools are basis of each of the examination activity in any research activity.

c. *Udaharana* (Example/Illustration) - The *udaharana* or example is the illustration that makes the more intelligent and the lesser understand a subject or topic with ease. This point again demonstrates the proximity of the science and society in the ancient period. The *udaharana* is the extension of the knowledge of the subject known to the unknown.

d. *Upanaya* (Discussion/Correlation) - The logical correlation of the data is studied under the umbrella of the *Upanaya*. The experimental data is correlated logically to the point of study. In general terms it can be better placed under the heading of logical discussion.

e. *Nigamana* (Conclusion) – The final word or the conclusion is the result of the research activity. It implies the acceptance or rejection of the hypothesis.

The last four points i.e. from *hetu* to the *nigamana* have been placed as the *sthapana* i.e. the justification of the hypothesis. Thus these four points are the tools of justification or validation of the asserted hypothesis.

Principles of discussion/teaching methodology:

The *Ayurveda* teaching methodology is a question of debate amongst the academicians as there is a view supporting the classical method of *Ayurveda* teaching while the others favour a contemporary subject specific study. The *Vimana Sthana* discusses the teaching methodology in *Ayurveda*. The *Vimana Sthana* describes the three methods of learning *Ayurveda* viz the *adhyayana* (studying), *adhyapana* (teaching) and *tadvidya sambhasha* (discussion with the like). There are 44 points of discussion known as the *vada marga*. These points of discussion include all the points of positive and healthy discussion that was the methodology of learning and knowledge exchange. The logical points of support in one's view and its counter augment of refute was the method adopted in that period. Finally the view that is logical and stands till end was accepted by all. Thus these ways of discussion was also a tool of learning.

The modern concepts of the seminars, symposia and the continued medical education programmes, CMEs are the modified version of the learning methodology described in the *Ayurveda* classical texts.

The teaching methodology explained in the *Vimana Sthana* is also unique as it gives an idea of the highest standards of teaching. The teacher has to prove his worth through the various points of *acharya pariksha*. The teacher compulsorily examines the worth of the student aspiring to be a physician. There are detailed rules and regulations of teaching and learning. This comprises of the special reference to the medical ethics to be strictly followed by the aspiring physician. The concept of the examination of the text to be studied is also explained under the heading *shastra pariksha*. Thus, the *Vimana Sthana* details the ideal teaching and learning methodology that is sufficient to produce the desired physicians which are a boon for the society.

Chapter 4

Vimana Sthana – The *Pariksha Sthana*

The *Vimana Sthana* of the *Charaka Samhita* is termed here as the *pariksha Sthana* i.e. the section of examinations. The *pariksha* means the *jijnasa* (desire). The desire to know something propels a person towards the examination. This goes in line with the adage 'Necessity is the mother of invention'. The necessity or yearning for something is the driving force or the guiding principle for the conduction of *pariksha* or examination. The *Vimana Sthana* is the knowledge unit and the knowledge is not attained without the examination. That is the reason why the seers of yore have put *pariksha* or examination under the umbrella of the *jijnasa*.

Jijnasa naama pariksha (*Charaka Samhita Vimana Sthana Chapter 8/46*)

The concept of *pariksha* originates from the Indian philosophical school of *Nyaya* well known for its detailed description of the means of true/valid enquiry known as *Pramana*. The systematic study of these tools of scientific enquiry is termed as 'Epistemology'. The epistemology or the *Pramana Vijnana* is the foundation stone of the development of the *Ayurveda* principles. The fourfold means of validation described in the Indian Philosophy of *Nyaya* viz. the *Pratyaksha* (direct observation/perception), *Anumana* (inference), *Shabda* (authoritative testimony) and *Upamana* (analogy) find their application in *Ayurveda* ubiquitously. The *Charaka Samhita* clearly explains the importance of the examination as the one that ultimately leads to the truth or the exact nature of the subject concerned. The *Sutra Sthana* of the *Charaka Samhita* chapter 11 namely the *Tisraishniyam Adhyaya* presents an in-depth description of the four tools with the addition of *yukti* (logic) in place of the *upamana* (analogy). It is however significant to note that the same classic mentions the *upamana* as one of the *hetu* (causative factors of cognition) in the chapter 8 of the *Vimana Sthana*. Therefore in fact *Charaka* also approves of the analogy as a tool of understanding and examination.

The aim of *pariksha* is the *pratippati jnana*. As stated by seer *Charaka*:

Parikshaayaastu khalu prayojanam pratipattijnaanam

(Charaka Samhita Vimana Sthana Chapter 8/132)

Pratipatti means the knowledge of the attributes as described by the seers in the classics like the knowledge of the disease and treatment.

The *pariksha* is also the synonym of research. The research also aims at the upgradation of knowledge possible through the examination. The *Vimana Sthana* of the *Charaka Samhita* presents the following examinations:

1. **Examination of the specific entities** - The *Vimana Sthana* of the *Charaka Samhita* presents the knowledge of the specific attributes necessary to know for the *Ayurveda* physician. These special attributes are the *dosha, dushya, rasa et al*. The knowledge of the *doshadi* is essential for a physician as without their knowledge the physician cannot think about the treatment. The measurement of these entities ensures a rational approach towards the diagnosis and treatment. The *Vimana Sthana* presents a detailed examination of these entities. The first chapter of the *Vimana Sthana* presents the concept of *prabhava* (special effect) in terms of the *dosha prabhava, rasa prabhava* important to be well understood by the aspiring physician. Without the knowledge of the measurement of these entities through their valid examination, the logic cannot be applied. The concept of the *prakriti samsamveta* (effect on

expected lines based on the constitution/composition) & *vikriti vishamasamveta* (deviation in the effect from expected lines based on its unique constitution/composition) is a guiding principle for the assessment of the drug effect or the manifestation of the disease.

2. **Examination of the food in terms of utility and quantity** – the food forms the base of the body. The *Ayurveda* physiology revolves around the food as the cause of the origin, growth and development of the living body. Even the disease is said to be caused because of the food, if not consumed as per the *Ayurveda* principles of intake and digestion. The *Vimana Sthana* details the food in terms of its composition taste (*rasa*) and the *ahara vidhi visheshayatana* (factors affecting the food intake and digestion). These eight factors have to be thoroughly understood in this era of junk and packed food. These eight factors namely the *prakriti* (natural constitution of the food), *karana* (processing), *samyoga* (combination), *rashi* (amount/diet), *desha* (place of origin and consumption), *kala* (time), *upayoga samstha* (rules of intake) and *upyokta* (user/consumer) are to be properly examined for the delivery of expected results. The food which is light i.e. having the dominance of the *vayu & agni mahabhuta* will be digested in less time due to its conduciveness with *agni*, the digestive fire as compared to the *guru* (heavy) food which gets digested in longer duration. Therefore the quantity of the food depends on the quality of the food i.e. the heavy food is to be taken half of the satiety level while the light food up to the satiety. The *Vimana Sthana* presents a hypothetical division of the capacity of the *kukshi* (stomach) into parts i.e. one part for the solid, the other part for the liquids and the last part to be left vacant for the *doshas*. Thus, it is

desirable to follow this rule as any shortcoming shall give birth to the causative factor of all the diseases which is known as *ama,* the improperly transformed food. This undesired product is said to be the cause of diseases thereby giving the name *áamaya* to the disease. This examination of the food assumes importance in the chapter 8 of the *Vimana Sthana* as well as *Charaka* presents the examination of the *ahara shakti* (food capacity) in terms of the ingestion and the digestion capacity.

3. **Examination of the natural factors like the air, water *et al.*** – The *Vimana Sthana* presents a subject of contemporary relevance in the name of the *janapadodhwamsa* (epidemics). The epidemics in *Ayurveda* philosophy is caused due to the vitiation of common natural factors of the *vayu* (air), *jala* (water), *desha* (region/habitat/land) and *kala* (time). These four factors are vitiated by the unchecked exploitation of the resources resulting out of the greed of the mankind termed as *adharma*. The examination of these four factors has been explained in the *Vimana Sthana*. The points of examination of these natural factors is summarized below-

Name of the factor	Normal characteristics	Vitiated Characteristics (compared with pollution)
Vayu (Air)	Conducive to the season i.e. having the properties in accordance with the concerned season, normal in speed, bearing the life, odourless, not inflated with the poisonous or foreign	Deviation from the season, excess of or loss of speed, and excess of dryness, coldness, hotness, roughness and humidity, and causing the cyclones and having stinky odour, appearance, sand and ash. These

	material.	characteristics are compared with the contemporary concept of air pollution mainly in the cities.
Jala (Water)	Tasteless, colourless, odourless, life of the living beings, normal specific gravity and viscosity	Taste, colour, odour – according to the pollutant, change in the specific gravity and viscosity, leads to the death of the dependent creatures i.e. destroys the marine ecosystem. The poisonous effluents from the factories and sewage drains are the major cause of the water pollution today.
Desha (Land/Region)	Soil is in accordance with the region with the expected flora & fauna flourishing. Pleasant and conducive living environment.	Soil is vitiated or polluted having the abnormal colour, smell, taste and touch, and full of unexpected animals in the particular region like the scavengers, mosquitoes, serpents, flies *et al.* The land having excessive dryness or wetness and is smoky. The skies are also not clear and give an unpleasant appearance.
Kala (Time)	The normal state of the seasons.	The seasons have a deviated look i.e. the weather conditions are not in line with the season. Like the rain in winter and the dry

	spells in the rainy season. The weather shows either excess, below normal or deviated weather termed as the *atiyoga, ayoga & mithya yoga.*

4. **Examination of the life span** – The life span of an individual is a question of debate as some believe it to be fixed while the others accept it to be fluctuating. The *ayu* in *Ayurveda* symbolize the life span. The *sutra Sthana* presents two definitions of *ayu*. *Ayu* is defined as the continuity of life and as the combination of the body, senses, mental entity and the aliveness (soul). The *Ayurveda* discusses the *ayu* in pragmatic way. The life-span depends upon the balance of the pre-determined *(daiva)* and the gained through visible effort *(purushkara)*. The actions done in the past life are the pre-determined while the actions done in this life are called the *purushkara.* These actions done are categorized as the mild, moderate and the strong. When the actions of the predetermined *daiva* and the cognizable, *purushkara* are of the strong category, the life-span is said to be long. If however, the actions of the two are of mild variety, the life span is less and in the case of the moderate actions the stronger of the two decides the fate of life-span. Therefore it is advisable to perform good deeds so that the life-span is longer and happy. The rejuvenating therapy is believed to act in the cases of fluctuating life span. The fixed life span cannot be extended and thus the rejuvenating therapy is futile in this case.

5. **Specific examination of the diseases** – The *Vimana Sthana* presents a detailed methodology of the diagnosis of disease in *Ayurveda*. The chapter 4 namely the *trividharoga vishesha vijnaniya adhyaya* is a treasure trove for the *Ayurveda* diagnostic tools. The three specific tools of examination of a disease are the *pratyaksha* i.e. direct observation through the senses, *anumana* (logical inference) and the classical testimony namely the *aptopadesha*. These three are collectively termed as *trividha jnana samudaaya,* the triad of knowledge.

6. **Examination of the *Srotasa* (channels)** – The unique basic principle of the disease and treatment in *Ayurveda* is the *srotasa* or the channel. The *srotasa* have been defined as those which carry the *dhatus*/tissues undergoing transformation. This is a very significant definition as it *per se* explains the role of the *srotasa* in nutrition (healthy state) and in the propagation of disease (vitiated state). The *Vimana Sthana* of the *Charaka Samhita* chapter five namely the *Sroto vimana Adhyaya* explains in detail the concept of *srotasa*. The thirteen varieties of the channels have been elaborated in regards to their origins, normal and abnormal functions with their cause of vitiation and thereafter the treatment protocol. This chapter forms the base of the *Ayurveda* diagnosis and treatment as the *Vimana Sthana* confirms to the compulsory involvement of the *srotasa* in the health and disease. The examination of these *srotasa* is invariably needed for the assessment of the pathogenesis (*samprapti*) of a disease. The propagation of the *dosha* is through the *srotasa* and the manifestation of the signs and symptoms also depends upon the status of the *srotasa* involved.

7. **Examination of the inner and external strength of the patient** – The *Vimana Sthana* again proves it's might as it presents the minute examination of the inner and external strength of the patient as an essential part of the examination. A mere examination of the compactness and physical appearance may mislead a physician regarding the overall strength of a patient, thereby rendering the physician to commit mistakes in deciding the line of treatment. The examination of the patient in all aspects is the key for correct assessment of a disease and the dosage of the drug. The dosage and the type of prescription is based upon the inner and external strength of the patient as it signifies the endurance capacity, an essential aspect of the examination.
8. **Examination of the body parasites/worms** – The chapter seven of the *Vimana Sthana* of *Charaka Samhita* is known for its in-depth description of the body parasite/worms likened with modern day parasitological deliberations. Some of the *Ayurveda* scholars have considered this description as an acceptance of the concept of the microorganisms in *Ayurveda*. The concept of the *raktaja krimi* has been particularly equated with the disease causing microorganisms. The *raktaja krimi* are said to be *adrishya* (invisible), *anu* (minute/tiny) *et al.* This chapter proposes the *saptaka gana* (examination of the seven tenets) including the *samutthana* (special cause), *Sthana* (habitat), *sanSthana* (form/appearance), *varna* (colour), *naama* (nomenclature), *prabhaava* (special effects), and the *chikitsa vishesha* (specific treatment). Although, these seven points of examination have been described in context of the *krimi* (parasite/worms), these are in-fact the general aspect of examination of any disease.

9. **Examination of the eligibility of the text, teacher and the student** – There has been a lot of debate regarding the ideal teaching and learning methodology in *Ayurveda* science. The *Vimana Sthana* being a knowledge and measurement unit brings to light the teaching methodology in *Ayurveda* and the foremost importance of ethical medical education. The ultimate chapter of the *Vimana Sthana* namely the *Rogabhishagjitiyam Adhyaya* elaborates the examination of the three basic aspects of teaching namely the teacher, the text and the pupil. Thus, *Ayurveda* proposes a perfection of these three to achieve the desired target of producing a quality physician which is a boon to the society and mankind. The chapter proposes the essential examinations of the three pillars of education. No other science has ever proposed such a rationale for the quality education. The salient points of examination of the teacher, text and the pupil are enumerated below:

   a. **The examination of text-** The points of examination of the text include the credibility of the author, the recommendation of the knowledgeable, free of the fallacies of repetitions, systematic presentation, easy to comprehend and full of illustrations.
   b. **The examination of teacher-** An ideal teacher should be sound in theoretical and practical knowledge, skilled, respectable, loving and caring for the pupil, dedicated and positive character.
   c. **The examination of pupil/student-** The student aspiring to be an *Ayurveda* physician should be examined in regards to his credentials, behaviour and patience, clear vision, intelligence, activity, generosity and obedience.

   These qualities make the student eligible for attaining the highest level of education through the ideal preceptor. The pupil therefore attains the oratory acumen along with the everlasting knowledge of the eternal science of *Ayurveda*.

Along with these examinations, the *Vimana Sthana* also proposes the methods of attaining knowledge namely the learning, teaching and the wise discussions. These three are the pillars of education.

10. **Examination of the amelioration/cure of the disease** – The philosophy of *Ayurveda* science is unique as it doesn't consider the mere cure/disappearance of disease as the health. The complete cure of a disease is the target of the *Ayurveda* treatment which is characterized by the alleviation of the pain, restoration of the voice and complexion, nourishment of the body, augmentation of the strength, desire to ingest and the digestion of the ingested, proper sleep and awakening, expulsion of the metabolic wastes. This is a major difference between the modern allopathic science of medicine and *Ayurveda*. Furthermore, the *Ayurveda* system postulates the attainment of *sukha* (happiness) characterized by the attainment of the state of satisfaction/pleasure of the mental unit, intellect, senses and the physical body. Thus, the *Ayurveda* aims at the achievement of a complete state of the restoration of the body and mind.

11. **Examination of the habitat** - The *Vimana Sthana* of the *Charaka Samhita* ponders over the examination of the *desha* (habitat) as an essential part of the routine examination. The *desha* is the *adhiSthana* (abode/substratum). This implies the region as well as the site of the health & disease, the human body. This again is quintessential example of holistic approach of the *Ayurveda* system of medicine. The region or the habitat involves the place of the birth, growth and development of a person or the medicine as the local climatic conditions affect the lifestyle of the person

and also affect the qualities of the plant products viz. the food and the medicine. The *desha* is thus the factor that affects the *bala* (strength) of the medicine and an individual. It is a common factor of the health and disease affecting a large number of people. The contemporary system of medicine also approves of the importance of the habitat as this affects the health of an individual. The people living in the African continent are more prone to the malaria parasite as compared to other continents while the people in the Indian Subcontinent are more susceptible to the tuberculosis than the European or American Diaspora. The people hailing from the state of Punjab and Arid regions of Rajasthan are naturally stronger as compared to the people of Gujarat or Madhya Pradesh. The place of one's dwelling is an important indication about the strata of living and thus the susceptibility towards a disease condition. *Ayurveda* again classifies the region as the *jangala* (dry/arid/scanty rainfall and vegetation), *anoopa* (wet/plenty of rainfall and vegetation) and the *sadharana* (moderate). These regions have been related to the status of the *dosha* as the *jangala* is *Vata* dominant, *anoopa* is *Kapha* dominant and the *sadharana* is conducive to all *dosha*. The *Ayurveda* considers the human body as a *desha* which needs to be taken care of through the *Ayurveda* dietary and other regimen prescribed in the classics. The deviation from the *Ayurveda* lifestyle leads to the diseases which again require the examination of the body in totality. These ten points of examination bring about a clear picture of the status of the body in regards to the strength and life-span (*ayu*).

12. **Examination of the natural constitution (*Prakriti*)** - The concept of *prakriti* is a basic concept of *Ayurveda*. The *prakriti* means nature which is unchangeable. It is the natural predisposition of the *dosha,* the mildly

increased state of the *dosha* which is acceptable to the body by the virtue of birth. The *dosha prakriti* is decided during the time of the fertization per se. The dominance of a *dosha* or a combination of *dosha* in the *shukra* (sperm/semen) & *shonita* (ovum) is manifested as the *prakriti*. The *prakriti* in-fact makes a person susceptible towards a disease/condition. The *vata prakriti* persons are more prone to have the *vata* diseases and *pitta* towards the *pitta* disorders *et al*. The significant contribution of the *Vimana Sthana* in this concept of *prakriti* is the description in terms of the *guna*/attribute of the *dosha*. The important features of the *dosha prakriti* in terms of the *dosha guna* are tabulated below.

Dosha	Attribute/Quality	Characteristic feature
Vata	*Rooksha* (dry)	*Rooksha* (dry), *apachita* (emaciated), *alpa* (dwarf) *shareera* (body) i.e. the people predominantly *vata* are less in physical built. Possess unattractive/unpleasant voice and are alert.
	Laghu (light)	Light and inconsistent gait. Incoherent action, food habits and movement
	Chala (mobile)	Instability in movement of head, shoulder, eyes, hands & legs.
	Bahu (plenty/ample)	Talkative, prominent tendons and veins
	Sheeghra (fast/swift)	Quick initiation and irritation, good grasping but weak memory, easily

		prone to attachment-detachment, fear *et al*.
	Sheeta (cool)	Intolerance to cold, easily afflicted with cold, stiffness and shivering (in cold conditions)
	Parusha (rough)	Roughness in the body parts
	Vishada (clear/non-slimy)	Cracking of the joints (less lubrication)
Pitta	*Ushna* (hot)	Intolerance to heat, warm mouth, delicate and fair body, plenty of skin eruptions like the moles, discolouration *et al*, early greying and falling of hair, early wrinkling of the skin and characteristic less, brown and soft scalp and body hair.
	Teekshna (quick/sharp)	Valour, brave, strong digestive fire, ravenous and thirsty, intolerance to disputes, frequent eaters
	Drava (fluid)	Soft and loose joints & muscles, abundant excretion of the sweat, urine and faeces
	Visra (foul odour)	Foul odour of the axilla, mouth, head and body
	Amla (sour) & *Katu* (pungent) tastes	Inadequate semen, sexual longing and procreation. Thus, the *pitta* dominant people are moderate.
Kapha	*Snigdha* (unctuous)	Unctuous organs i.e. are not dry

		(compared from *vata prakriti*)
	Slakshna (smooth)	Smoothness in the normally smooth organs/units like the nails
	Mridu (soft)	Pleasant/attractive appearance, delicate and fair body
	Madhura (sweet)	Abundance of the semen, sexual activity and progeny.
	Saara (concrete)	Firm, compact and stable body
	Saandra (dense)	Well developed and complete body
	Manda (slow)	Slow in action and other activities
	Stimita (unwavering)	Slow initiators and high bearing people
	Guru (heavy)	Confident and stable gait
	Sheeta (cool)	Lesser hunger, thirst, heat and sweat
	Vijjala (thick)	Joints and their ligaments compact
	Accha (lucid)	Happy and joyful presentation

These characteristics of the *prakriti* in accordance with the attributes of the *guna* of the constituent *dosha* is very practical manner of the ascertainment of *prakriti* and is helpful in deciding the conducive regimen for an individual in regards to the seasonal and diurnal variations. The *guna* play the most important part in the choice of a *dravya* suitable to the needs of an individual.

13. **Examination of the *dhatu* excellence** – *Saara* is the best quality of the tissue/*dhatu*. To assess the status of the tissue in regards to its strength and weakness, the *saara* becomes an important part of the clinical examination. The eight varieties of *saara* on the basis of the quality of the

tissue are assessed as the best (*pravara*), medium (*madhyama*) and the low (*avara*). The examination of the *dhatus* is based upon the signs and symptoms mentioned in the classics especially the *Vimana Sthana* of the *Charaka Samhita* chapter eight namely the *rogbhishagjitiya adhyaya*. These signs are of great significance particularly for the poor states as they are the alternate arrangement of the assessment of the tissues without any help from the costly laboratory tests. However, it is essential to have a research to translate these subjective parameters to the objective ones so that a uniform scientific standard may be set. Some common ailments affecting vast areas of the third and underdeveloped world can be easily diagnosed through these parameters. These characteristics are a result of careful observation by the seers of yore postulated for the benefit of mankind. Some of the unique observations observed by the seers especially the *Charaka* are-

a. Observation of the teeth for the assessment of the status of the semen (*shukra*). *Charaka Samhita* postulates that the person with the best quality of the *shukra* is characterized by the systematic alignment and excellent appearance of the teeth.

b. The observation of the status of the plasma (*rasa*) is through the examination of the skin. The soft and shiny skin with soft and scanty body hair suggests the good status of the *rasa*.

c. The examination of the status of the mind is through the level of confidence. The ability of bear the extremes in life is suggestive of the best mental strength.

14. **Examination of the body size** – The *pramana* is one of the ten-fold examinations of the strength of an individual. Here the seer *Charaka*

utilizes the various aspects of measurement like the length, breadth and the measurement of capacity in term of the *anjali pramana* of the liquid/semi-solid body units like the *rasa, rakta, meda, mutra et al*. The ideal body size is supposed to be of 84 *angula* (finger breadth) of the concerned person. The measurement of the vital body parts which are vulnerable to injury and commonly known as *marma* in *Ayurveda* parlance has been clearly described. These parts are to be taken care of while performing any *shalya* procedure like the cautery or surgery.

15. **Examination of the homologation/adaptability** – This concept of homologation or adaptability is again a fundamental principle of the *Ayurveda* system of medicine. This has been termed as the *saatmya* in *Ayurveda* terminology. The *saatmya* refers to the homologation of the body to a particular thing/entity on prolonged exposure. This concept is utilized in the maintenance of health and treatment of the disease. The *Ayurveda* advises the homologation for all the six tastes (*shad rasa*) as a key factor for the health maintenance. Likewise, the food items which are homologous since birth are the ghee, milk, and honey *et al*. The seer cautions the consumer about the long term harmful effect of the homologation of the non-beneficial. The seer again pragmatically mentions the sequential renunciation of the non-beneficial homologation through the sequential consumption/intake of the beneficial.

Therefore, this chapter ponders over the types of examination which are the crux of discussion in the *Vimana Sthana* of the *Charaka Samhita*. The *Vimana Sthana* of *Charaka Samhita* therefore has been considered here as a *pariksha Sthana*. The examinations mentioned in the *Vimana Sthana* have wide range of implications in expanding the theoretical as well as practical skill of an aspiring *Ayurveda* academician and a practitioner.

Chapter 5

Vimana Sthana of *Charaka Samhita* - Applied aspect

The *Vimana Sthana* of the *Charaka Samhita* presents an opportunity for the *Ayurveda* scholars to progress further in terms of development of the *Ayurveda* theory and clinical skills as it forms the base of the research protocol in *Ayurveda*. This chapter shall look into the various applications of the *Vimana Sthana* towards the maintenance of the health of the healthy and the best treatment for the ailing mankind, the two aims of the *Ayurveda* science.

The curative aspect of *Ayurveda* is of prime importance from the ancient times when only it was the system of medicine particularly in India. In the clinical practice, the two types of people seek an opinion of the physician viz. the ones longing for the maintenance of health while the others seeking the medical intervention for their ailments. Thus this chapter aims to bring to light the applied aspect of the *Vimana Sthana* of *Charaka Samhita* in terms of the two aims of *Ayurveda*.

Vimana Sthana & *the Swasthasya Swasthyarakshana:*

The first aim of the *Ayurveda* philosophy is to maintain the health of the healthy. This is achieved by the following of the *Ayurveda* deliberations on the maintenance of health. This covers the broad aspect of dietetics and the following of the regimen. The *Ayurveda* being a holistic system of medicine forms a balance between the microcosm, man and the macrocosm, environment. All the ways of the maintenance of health are in tandem with the natural variations like that of the season and the time. The specific regimen for every season according to the climatic conditions as well as their manifestations in the body has been carefully described. The variation in the time, seasons and movement of the sun affects the body parameters within normal limits. The *dosha* also show their normal increase in accordance with the movement of the sun. The *Vimana Sthana* presents the concept of the eight primary factors of food under the heading of the *ashta aahaara vidhi visheshayatana*. These eight factors along with the deliberations on the special effects i.e. *prabhaava* like the *rasa prabhaava* have an important role in the maintenance of the state of health. The food in *Ayurveda* is one of the three *upastambha* (supporting pillars) necessary to maintain the three primary pillars namely the *tridosha*. The *Vimana Sthana* deliberates upon the wholesome regimen as an essential part of the daily routine. The eight factors of food can be grouped as the *pathya* (beneficial) for the body. The equilibrium of the *dosha* is maintained through a careful ingestion of the six *rasas*. The *prakriti sam samaveta* & the *vikriti vishama samaveta* is a significant contribution of the *Vimana Sthana* of *Charaka Samhita*. This helps in the assessment of the action of the food and its composition. The special effect of some of the drugs/food is attributed to the unique combination of the *panchmahabhuta* (five basic elements) while the actions according to the expectations is attributed to the normal combination of the *panchmahabhuta*.

The *Vimana Sthana* also mentions in detail the method of food intake as the *aahaara vidhi vidhana* which is of significant relevance today. The methodology of the food intake has its corresponding effect on the digestive fire (*agni*). Today in many ways people have greater opportunities of better life than ever before. The scientific and economic developments have ensured the availability of the electronic gadjets which are being overused by the people. Even while having their food, the full concentration is towards these instruments thus rendering the consumer to eat more than what is sufficient. The dietetics is one of the most important factors of life. In this era of modernization and civilization, although the society is conscious enough about "What to eat or what not to eat", inspite of the awareness about the food items, their quantity, quality and nutritional values, the people are indulging into the excessive comsumption of the packed and instant foods. This can be understood as the intellectual blasphemy or the *prajnaparadha*. The dietetic code or the rules for diet intake are preserved by our traditions upto some extent, but there is a big question about their careful following. Thus, it becomes mandatory to follow the rules of dietary intake, *Ahara Vidhi Vidhana*. For the *swasthya rakshana*, the food is the most important factor. It when comsumed properly in accordance with the principles of *Ayurveda* leads to the augmentation of the strength, complexion and proper development & growth. On the contrary, proper diet if not taken in proper manner is a leading cause of diseases. The underdeveloped world faces the problem of malnourishment and starvation while the developed world faces the problem of over-eating leading to the obesity.

The dietetic code includes the principles of:

1. **Consumption of food afresh (*Ushanam*)** - The qualities that are achieved by taking freshly prepared (hot/warm) food are proper and timely digestion along with the maintenance of optimum taste, beneficial for the maintenance of the health. The *Ayurveda* thus prohibits the stale food as validated by the modern sciences as the more time renders the food liable for decay and putrifaction.

2. **Unctuous food (*Snigdham*)** - Unctuous (*Snigdha*) does not necessarily mean the oily substances but the food which is beneficial for the control of *vata* & *pitta* along with an optimum increase of *kapha*. The continuous and prolonged consumption of the dry (*ruksha*) food causes the weakness of the body and lessens the immunity as it is the prime cause of the rise of *vata*.

3. Optimum quantitity (*Maatraavat*) -

Food taken in optimum quantity is called as *Maatraavat*. *Ayurveda* approves the uniqueness of evry human and thus the optimum quantity of food and medicine cannot be fixed. Therefore the quantity of food depends upon ones own digestion power or the *agni*. *Ayurveda* approves of the two types of the food quantity i.e. the *sarvagraha & parigraha*. The *sarvagraha* means the total diet i.e. it includes all the nutrients taken together while the *parigraha* signifies of the quantity specific to the nutrients. The two methods of calculation of the quantity of food are to be examined in regards of the *prakriti, vayah, karma & agni*. The optimum quantity of the food is that which does not lead to the diseases of digestion and is timely digested.

4. **Proper time of food intake (*jeerne*)** – A person aspiring to be healthy should ingest the food only after the digestion of the previous food. This leads to the maintenance of the *doshas* and thereby promotes the life.

5. **Compatible food intake (*Veerya aviruddham*)** – The food articles to be consumed should be compatible to ones body. A person should avoid the food which is antagonistic to the body tissues termed broadly as the *viruddha aahaara*. Apart from being compatible, the food to be consumed should be having the desired nutrients i.e. potency. The potency (*veerya*) is an important quality a substance as it is the one that renders activity to a substance.

6. **Conducive/pleasant environment (*ishte deshe*)** – The *Vimana Sthana* of the *Charaka Samhita* mandates the ingestion of the food in the conducive environment or a congenial place having all the necessary accessories for pleasurable feeling as the sound psychological condition supports the digestion of the food. The unpleasant dining area decreases the *agni* as it afflicts the mind.

In the current scenario, this suitable place should be properly understood as perfectly clean and hygienic.

7. **Availability of all the necessary accessories (*ishta sarvopakaranam*)** - Appropriate necessary appliances/instruments for dining include the clean utensils required for preparation, serving, storage and dining of food. This again bestows a pleasurable feeling in a person thereby promoting digestion.

8. **Patient dining (*Na atidrutam - Na ativilambitam*)** - The food should not be eaten in a rush. The hurried consumption may make the food enter into the other pathway like the breathing path. The haste in eating the food makes a person insensitive towards the quality of food and thus the desired effects cannot be achieved. On the contrary, food should not be eaten too leisurely/slowly as it leads to overeating and thereby obesity and indigestion. Therefore, the food should be consumed in a manner neither too fast nor too slow.

9. **Concentrated and sensitive dining (*Ajalpana, ahasana, tanmana bhunjita*)** – The food should be eaten with full concentration. The laughing or talking while the consumption of food makes a person suffer from the problems of indigestion or that associated with the hastily consumption of food. To attain the optimum benefit of the food, it needs to be eaten with full and complete concentration.

Thus the *Ayurveda* system of medicine takes utmost care about the food habits and the *Vimana Sthana* of *Charaka Samhita* presents an excellent deliberation on the methodology of food intake and its benefits.

Deliberations on the *aahaara maatraa* (quantity of food) –

The dietetic code in the *Vimana Sthana* of the *Charaka Samhita* consists of a clear view on the quantity of the food in accordance to ones digestive power, *agni*. The concept of the wholesomeness and unwholesomeness of the diet with its merits and demerits has been well explained in the chapter two of the *Vimana Sthana* namely the *Trividhakuksheeya Vimana Adhyaya*.

Deliberations on the unity of the man & environment (the balancing act):

The unity of the man and the nature is very well depicted in the concept of the *Janapadodhwamsa* as the four common factors related to the nature viz. the air (*vaayu*), the water (*jala*), the place/region (*desha*) and the time (*kala*). This unity of the man and the nature is the hallmark of the *Ayurveda* system of medicine. The greed of the man for power and dominance leading to the war and unrest is considered to be the causative factor of the destruction of nature and thus the balance between the man and the environment gets disturbed leading to the epidemics. The harmony between the two is explained in terms of the judicious use of the natural resources and following the prescribed code of conduct.

Regimens for the four categories of people in accordance with the natural constitution (*prakriti*):

The *Vimana Sthana* of *Charaka Samhita* deliberates upon the means of remaining healthy for the four categories of people viz. *vatala, pittala, shleshmala* & the *sama dosha prakriti*. The *sama prakriti* person should follow the regimen that maintains the balance of the *dosha* while the *dosha* dominant constitutions like the *vatala, pittala & shleshmala* should follow the regimen which is antagonistic to the naturally increased/predominant *dosha*. Although, the deliberations on the natural physical constitution i.e. *prakriti* have been postulated in the *sootra Sthana* itself, the methodology to understand the *prakriti* and following of a beneficial regimen is enunciated in the *Vimana Sthana* of *Charaka Samhita*.

In this way, the *Vimana Sthana* of the *Charaka Samhita* is a complete section of *Ayurveda* dealing with both the issues of the maintenance of health and the treatment of the diseased.

Vimana Sthana & the Aturasya Vikara Prashamana:

The ultimate aim of the *Ayurveda* system of medicine is the treatment of the suffering mankind. The *Vimana Sthana* presents a deep insight into the methods of treatment including the systematic diagnosis as the latter is the cause of the proper and judicious treatment. The main points of the *Aturasya Vikara Prashamana* i.e. the curative aspect of the *Vimana Sthana* are described below:

Triad of the diagnostic *(naidaanika)*, curative *(chikitsya)*, and the beneficial/wholesome *(pathya)* aspect:

The complete system of *Ayurveda* philosophy of medicine includes the diagnosis, treatment and the attainment of normalcy through the strict adherence to the wholesomeness *(pathya)*. The patient when approaches a physician, it is becomes mandatory for the physician to diagnose the disease to perfection. The perfect and systematic diagnosis is based upon the complete clinical diagnostic methodology which is taken due care in the *Vimana Sthana*. The chapter four of the *Vimana Sthana* is a guiding tool for all the physicians as it deliberates upon the methodology of examination based on the tools proposed by the philosophers of yore. The main points of examination are tabulated below:

Tool of the examination	Name of the examination	Entities for examination
Pratyaksa (Direct observation)	Śrotendriya Prātyakṣa (auditory perception)	- Borborygmies - crepitus sound in the joints - heart and lung sounds - characteristic voices
	Cakṣurendriya Prātyaksa (visual perception)	- complexion - appearance, size & shape - shadow - normal features and the abnormalities of body - All the visual subjects of the body.
	Sparśendriya Prātyaksa (tactile perception)	- Normal and abnormal tactile sensations
	Ghrāṇendriya Prātyaksa (olfactory perception)	- standard and abnormal odour
	Rasanendriya Prātyaksa (Gustatory perception)	Cannot be perveived directly (known through inference)
Anumana (Inference)	Agni (Digestive fire)	Jaraṇa śakti (Strength of digestion)
	Bala (Strength)	Vyāyāma śakti (Capacity for workouts)
	Indriya (Acuity of the	Capacity of perception of their

	Senses/organs)	objects
	Sāttvika Mana	Normal and virtuous actions/behavior
	Rājasika Mana	Over excitement/ attachments
Aptopadesha/Shabda (Authoritative statement)	All the classical knowledge/*Ayurveda Upadesha* about the methods of maintaining the health and also the diagnostics & treatment.	

Similarly, the essential point of the *Ayurveda* diagnosis of a disease is the channels of progression of a disease known as *srotasa* in *Ayurveda* parlance. The chapter five of the *Vimana Sthana* of *Charaka Samhita* vividly explains the characterstics of the healthy and the unhealthy state of various channels with their causative factors of vitiation. This is one of the most important features of the diagnosis of a disease.

The chapter six of the *Vimana Sthana* deliberates upon the types of the *agni,* the factor for transformation. The diseases are said to be caused by the vitiation of *agni* and thus the *Vimana Sthana* assists in the identification of the status of *agni*. This chapter also discusses upon the classification of the diseases and is the guiding principle for the nomenclature of the diseases hitherto absent from the *Ayurveda*.

Likewise the chapter eight of the *Vimana Sthana* is a treasure of *Ayurveda* knowledge as it presents an indepth description of the tenfold examination of diseased which can be considered as the mother of all the examination. These ten points cover almost all the aspects of an individual health and the disease and is the crème – de – la – crème in the diagnostic principles in the *Ayurveda* science of medicine.

***Vimana Sthana* - The Curative aspect:**

Coming to the curative aspect of the *Vimana Sthana* of the *Charaka Samhita*, it is quite clear that although the treatment protocol has been explained in the *chikitsa Sthana* (the section dealing with the treatment), the principles of treatment have been explicated in the *sootra Sthana* and thereafter the other sections including the *Vimana Sthana*.

The expositions on the curative aspect are explained herewith:

a. **The concept of *Aama* (improperly transformed entity especially the food & the tissues) and its management** – The fundamental concept of the *aama* is a unique *Ayurveda* principle. The beginning of all the diseases is attributed to this state thereby giving the name *aamaya* to the disease. The chapter two of the *Vimana Sthana* of *Charaka Samhita* namely the *Trividhakukshiya Adhyaya* deals with the concept of quantity of food in terms of its wholesomeness and non- wholesomeness and their effects on the body. The food taken in excess i.e. beyond the quantity that can be digested properly is the causativefactor for the *aama*. This *aama* is of two types namely the *Alasaka & Visuchikaa*. The chapter vividly explains the pathogenesis of these two states along with their treatment principle.

The treatment principle of the *alasaka* is the forceful expulsion of the accumulated *dosha* through the mouth i.e. the emesis by the warm saline solution. Followed by the emesis is the sudation, use of suppository and then the *langhana* (lightning therapy).

The *visuchikaa* is ameliorated through the *langhana* followed by the care taken for the person who has undergone purgation therapy.

In the context of the treatment of the *aama,* it has been explained that the main therapy is the *apatarpana* (emaciation therapy). Inspite of the application of the emaciation therapy if the *dosha* still persists then the line of treatment should be the *nimitta viparita* (against the causative factor). If this also fails then the treatment should be *aatanka viparita* i.e. specific treatment of a disease. This line of treatment is applied in a number of diseases like the *jwara, chhardi et.al.*

b. **The management of an epidemic (*janapadodhwansa*)** – The chapter three of the *Vimana Sthana* of *Charaka Samhita* details about the burning problem of the contemporary world i.e. the epidemics. The general line of treatment of the epidemic is the *panchkarma* (five fold therapy of purification) followed by the use of the *rasaayana* (antioxidants & tonics), preparation of the body through the potent drugs and ultimately a strict adherence to the ethical regimen prescribed in the classical texts. This also includes the harmony between the man and the environment which is the topic of discussion in the world today in the form of the climate change and greenhouse emissions.

c. **The management of the parasite/pathogens (*krimi chikitsa*)** – The management of the *krimi* (parasites and germs) has been enunciated in the *Charaka Samhita* perhaps for the first time in the *Ayurveda* classics. A detailed description of the types of the *krimi* with their effects on the body is avialble in the *Vimana Sthana*. The treatment of these parasites including the pathogens is three-fold as described below:

i. *Apakarshana* (Expulsion) – The first line of management for the parasites is their forceful purgation/expulsion from the body. This can be achieved through the manual pulling of the visible parasite or through the use of the purgative medicines. This method again, is a common practice of getting rid of the disturbing agent. The method followed is alike any other expulsion therapy. This consists of the *poorvakarma* i.e. the prior preparatory therapies of the oleation and the sudation followed by the application of the purgative therapy. The only difference is that prior to the purgation, the food/drugs promoting the growth or luring the parasites is used so as to facilitate their easy expulsion.

ii. *Prakritivighaata* (Anti-parasital drugs) – This implies the use of the drugs/diet which is non-conducive or against the nature of the *krimi*. This can be compared with the present day use of anthelmintics or vermicidal drugs. The seer *Charaka* has included the following drugs and diet under this section -

Moolakparni (Moringa oleifera) along with the red variety of rice, Oil of *Vidanga* (Embelia ribes), *Pippali* (Piper longum), *Chavya* (Piper chaba), *Chitraka* (Plumbago zeylanica), *Shrimgavera* (Zingiber officinale), *Nirgundi* (Vitex nigundo), *Kiraatatikta* (Swertia chirata) et al.

iii. *Nidaana Parivarjana* (Renunciation of the causative factor) - This principle is a universally approved principle in the *Ayurveda* system of medicine. The *nidaana* means the causative factor of a disease/entity. The simplest method of treatment is the avoidance of the causative factor. According to the theory of The

Swabhaavoparamavaada or the 'theory of destruction sans any cause'. The word *Swabhaava* means natural or innate and the *Uparama* means destruction/depletion. The physician's job is to ensure the production of the best *dhaatus* by strengthening the transformation factor of *Agni* followed by the dietary regimen. By doing so, the normal *dhaatus* will be produced and the vitiated ones naturally undergo the degradation as per the theory of *Swabhaavoparamavaada*. Thus, the renunciation of the causative factor of the production of *krimi* is a part of the treatment of the *krimi*.

d. **The management of the *dosha*-** The *Vimana Sthana* of the *Charaka Samhita* deals with the deliberations on the general management of *dosha*. The general mode of treatment of the three *dosha* viz. *vata, pitta & kapha* has been explained in the *Vimana Sthana*. This deliberation has been in the context of the *prakriti* but can be applied in all the treatment procedures of the *dosha*.

Thus the *Vimana Sthana* of *Charaka Samhita* is a complete section dealing with the diagnosis and treatment.

The *pathya* (wholesomeness) – In the *Ayurveda* system of medicine, the *pathya* i.e. the food and the actions that are beneficial to the body are considered to be most important. If the person is habitual to the wholesomeness of diet, there is no need for the medicine. Similarly the medicine becomes useless if not sufficed with the suitable *pathya*. The Pathya can be understood as the *Ashtau Ahaara Vidhi Visheshaayatanaani & Aahaara Vidhi Vidhaana* with the required modefications, if any.

The mere mitigation of the signs and symptom of a disease is not the target of *Ayurveda* treatment. The actual treatment means the restoration of the normalcy state i.e. the state prior to the disease manifestation. Once a disease is ameliorated, the wholesomeness of diet and other regimen aimed to increase the strength (*bala*) is advised as in the case of management of the *janapadodhwansa* & *aama vyadhi*. The word *patha* means the *srotasa/channel*. The details of the *srotasa* has been mentioned in the Vimana Sthana chapter 5 namely the *SrotoVimana Adhyaya*. So the regimen that is beneficial or wholesome for the channels and thus the body is said to be *pathya*. The seer advises the intake of the compatible diet (*aviruddha aahaara*). The compatible food is not against the tissues (*dhaatus*) and thus is beneficial for the body.

To summarize the applied aspect of the Vimana Sthana of the *Charaka* Samhita, it can be said beyond doubt that it makes the full complement if the preventive aspect followed by the deliberations on the appropriate treatment regimen in systematic manner. In continuation with the principles explained in the *sootra Sthana,* the Vimana Sthana clarifies and quantifies the knowledge of the basic principles of the *Ayurveda* science.

Chapter 6

Summary of the *Vimana Sthana* with its contemporary significance

The *Ayurveda* system of medicine is based on the fundamental principles having which are in the coded form mainly in the three great treatises namely the *Charaka Samhita, Sushruta Samhita* and the *Vagbhata Samhita*. The *Charaka Samhita* is the numero-uno treatise of the *Ayurveda* system of medicine. It acts as a guide for all the Ayurvedic practitioners and academicians. The seers have used their own particular style of narration in *Charaka Samhita* which needs to be understood properly to bring about the desired levels of the theoretical and practical know-how in the *Ayurveda* scholars. The *Charaka Samhita* is unique in many sorts as it presents a comprehensive view of *Ayurveda* system. Thus, it is termed as an *Ayurveda* encyclopaedia that is the guiding principle for understanding the classical approach as well as prospective of research activity in *Ayurveda*.

The Charaka Samhita has been rightly quoted as the *kalpadruma* by the revered commentator *Gangadhara Roy* in the commentary *Jalpakalpadruma*. The literary research of the *Charaka Samhita* also reveals its transformation at various levels of time. The *Charaka Samhita* is therefore the *Ayurveda* encyclopaedia that needs to be decoded in all its supremacy for the propagation and development of the *Ayurveda* system of medicine. Although the introduction to Charaka is difficult as some consider *Charaka* as an individual while the others consider him as a name of a group. Whatever the case may be, it is significant that the classical text available stands tall and verified to be scientific when doubted and subjected to the scientific examination.

Amongst the various sections of the *Charaka Samhita*, the *sootra Sthana* is the brain/head i.e. enjoys the topmost position in the text as it contains all the principles of the *Ayurveda* medicine in the coded form which need to be decoded. The principles in the *sootra Sthana* are valid elsewhere in the complete text.

The *Vimana Sthana* of the *Charaka Samhita* has been dealt with here as it is the knowledge and measurement unit. A science is incomplete without the measurement and complete knowledge. The *Vimana Sthana* gives us an opportunity to understand the *maana* (measurement units) of the essential components like the *dosha, dhaatu, et al.* Without the knowledge of the measurements, the science cannot progress further in light of the scientific parameters. The whole process of standardization is based on the concepts mentioned in the *Vimana Sthana*.

The number of verses/*Sootras* in the *Vimana Sthana* according to different authentic books/commentaries of the *Charaka Samhita* is tabulated below:

Name of the Chapter	No. of verses – Chakrapaani Dutta (*Ayurveda Deepikaa*)	No. of verses – Gangaadhara Roy (*Jalpakalpataru*)	No. of verses – Yogindranath Sen (*Charakopaskaara*)
Rasa Vimana	28	24	50
Trividhakukshiya Vimana	19	12	25
Janapadodhwamsaniya Vimana	52	27	56

Trividharogavishesha Vijnaniya Vimana	14	08	21
Sroto Vimana	31	09	46
Roganika Vimana	22	15	32
Vyadhitarupiya Vimana	32	17	33
Rogabhishagjitiya Vimana	157	127	190
Total	355	239	453

From the above table, it is clear that the three main commentaries on the *Charaka Samhita* vary in the context of numbering the verses. This is a unique way/style of description of a topic by a commentator. Some of the commentators comment upon some of the verses collectively thereby the numbers of verses seem to be decreased while actually they are not. On the other hand, the other seers comment upon them separately so that the number of verses seems to be more like that of the *Charakopaskaara* commentary of *Yogindranath Sen*. However it is noteworthy that there is no contradiction in principle which is desirable for the progression of a science.

The summary of all the eight chapters of the *Vimana Sthana* is mentioned below:

1. **The *Rasa Vimana*** – This chapter one of the *Vimana Sthana* begins with a deliberation on the meaning of the *Vimana* with its scope and utility. It has been said to be a measurement and a knowledge unit. The measurement termed as *maana* in *Ayurveda* parlance is established as the

cause of the standard diagnosis and treatment. In the beginning itself, there is a mention of ninefold examination viz. *dosha, bheshaja, desha, kala, bala, shareera, saara, aahaara, sattva, saatmya, prakriti* and *vaya*. Followed by these examinations, is the explanation of the special effect i.e. *prabhaava* of the combination of the *rasa, dosha* and *dravya*. A very significant concept of the *vikritivishamasamaveta* i.e. unique/differently constituted medicine/food is a key factor affecting the action of a substance. Some of substances are in harmony with their expected actions based on their constitution while the others act in an unexpected/unponderable manner. Thus giving rise to the special effect known as *prabhaava* in *Ayurveda*. The *rasaVimana* explains the special effect of the substances/*dravya* commonly used in the mitigation of the *pitta, vaata* and the *kapha* namely the *sarpi* (Ghee), *taila* (vegetable oils) and the *madhu* (honey). Similarly, the seer also cautions against the regular use of the three substances viz. *pippali (Piper longum), kshara (caustics/alkalis) & lavana (salt)*. The concept of conduciveness/harmony with the body known as *saatmya* has also been explained with its three categories namely the *pravara, madhyam and avara*. Followed by this is the vivid explanation of the concept of *ashta aahaara vidhi visheshaayatanaani* i.e. the deciding/governing factors for the beneficial/non-beneficial effect of the diet. Along with these eight factors, there is a significant deliberation on the manner of the food intake i.e. *aahaara vidhi vidhaana*.

In the contempory lifestyle of the superfast man, the food habits have totally changed as there is either an overeating or unhealthy eating or malnutrition and starvation. Thus, there is an ever increasing need to understand and propagate these golden principles of dietetics for availing the best and desired results.

2. **The *Trividhakuksheeya Vimana*** - This chapter is a continuous deliberation on the quantity of food, an important parameter necessary to be taken care of for the digestion and its subsequent results. The chapter presents a vivid description on the division of the *kukshi*/stomach into three parts for the ascertainment of proper digestion. It is infact a word of caution for the voracious eaters. A person desiring to gain the maximum nutrients from the food ingested i.e. proper digestion and assimilation, should ingest the food upto a two-third capacity (one third for the solids and the same for the liquid diet) of the stomach. The other third should be left empty for the movement of the *doshadi*. Followed by this, there is a subjective examination of the *maatraavat aahaara* (optimum amount of food) and *amaatraavat aahaara* (deviation from the optimum amount of food). The *amaatraavat aahaara* includes both i.e. the *ati- maatraa* (over - eating) and the *heena - maatraa* (under – eating). The over-eating is the causative factor of the disease condition known as the *aama* (the uncooked/untransformed intermediate product). This state is again manifested into two varieties namely the *alasaka* and *visoochikaa*. The chapter systematically explains the *alasaka & visoochikaa* along with its pathogenesis and treatment modality. This chapter has significant contribution in the three way treatment procedures namely the *hetu vipareeta* (anti-causative factor), *aatanka vipareeta* (anti-disease/specific), *ubhaya vipareeta* and *tadarthakaari chikitsaa* (anti - cause & disease, the favouring cause and disease). .

3. **The *Janapadodhwansaneeya Vimana*** – This chapter is specifically dedicated to the modern day epidemiology. The common factors affecting a group of population are the *vaaya, jala, desha* and *kala*. The *Vimana Sthana* presents an in-depth analysis of the wholesomeness of these four factors as the cause of health and *vice-versa*. This chapter can be understood in the modern light in terms of the pollution or ruthless exploitation of the natural resources. The world community is grappling with the serious issues of the climate change and its subsequent effects. The outbreak of epidemics in various parts of the globe is a frequently observed phenomenon having its root somewhere in the malptactices of the human beings. All these factors have been taken care of in this chapter along with its remedy.

4. **The *Trividharogavisheshavijnaaneeya Vimana*** – This chapter is base of the diagnosis in *Ayurveda* medical knowledge. The three basic principles of the diagnosis/examination of a disease are based on the three tools of examinations postulated in the Indian Philosophical schools mainly the *Nyaaya* system of *Gautama*. This three- fold methodology of examination includes the *Pratyaksa* (direct observation through the senses augmnented by the use of the modern aids like the microscope and stethoscope), the *Anumana* (logical inference based on the inherent relation between the cause and effect) and the *Aptopadesha/Shabda* (authoritative statement of the trustworthy). All the contemporary medical examinations fall under one of these three categories.

5. **The *Srotasaam Vimana*** – This chapter is the base of the *Ayurveda* basic principles of nutrition and transformation of various tissues in the healthy state. It also deliberates upon the propagation, manifestation, diagnosis

and treatment of a disease. The basic tubular structures called *Srotasa* (channels) have been explained in detail in regards to their normalcy and abmormality.

6. **The *Rogaaneeka Vimana*** – The *Rogaaneeka Vimana* deals with the basic principles of nomenclature of a disease hitherto unknown along with the vivid description of the factor of transformation in *Ayurveda* namely the *agni*. This basic factor has been defined in accordance with the *prakriti* or natural constitution of person. The chapter also presents a summary of the susceptibility of the single *dosha prakriki* towards their constituting *dosha* along with the treatment protocol.

7. **The *Vyadhitrupeeya Vimana*** - This chapter aims at the ascertaiment of the actual position of the disease and diseased based on the mental strength or will power of a patient. The two categories of patients have been explained, first with a strong mental composition bearing even the dreadful conditions and making the serious condition look moderate while the other category having a weak mental composition not bearing even the moderate conditions and making them appear serious. Thus, this misleading concept must be clarified as the treatment (especially the dosage and choice of therapy) depends upon the pinpoint diagnosis. This chapter details about the *krimi* compared with the present day parasitology including the micro-organisms compared with the *raktaja krimi*. The three-fold treatment modality namely the *apakarshana* (expulsion), *prakritivighaata* (anti parasites) and the *nidaana parivarjana* (renunciation of the cause).

8. **The *Rogbhishagjiteeya Vimana*** - This chapter aims to create a clear vision of the *Ayurveda* methodology of teaching and learning. This

chapter forms the base of the research methodology in Ayurveda. The tenfold points of examination called the *dashavidha pareekshya bhaava* are the base of research methodology. Similarly the threefold methods of increasing the knowledge or the *jnaanopaaya* are the learning, teaching, and the seminars/discussions. The chapter presents a detailed view of these methods with their eligibility criteria along with the forty-two points of discussion under the umbrella of the *vaada maarga*. The detailed explanation of the *prakriti* in terms of the *guna* (attribute) is a great contribution of the *Charaka Samhita* and the *Vimana Sthana*. The chapter also presents the *aushadha pariksha* (points of drug research) in the context of *karana* (instrument/tool). The *dashavidha parikshaa* (tenfold) examination of the patient is the best diagnostic tool in *Ayurveda* medicine. The ten points of examination include all the parameters to be considered for a correct assessment of the strength of a partient and the diagnosis of a disease. This chapter thus is a treasure trove of the basic principles of *Ayurveda* education and learning with the fundamentals of research.

To summarize the *Vimana Sthana*, it can be said that:

a. It is a *parikshaa Sthana* (section of examinations)
b. Is a knowledge unit
c. Is a measurement unit
d. Is a base for research
e. Is a base for *Ayurveda* education and learning

REFERENCES/BIBLIOGRAPHY

CLASSICAL TEXTS

- *Sushruta Samhita* (*Sootra Sthana*) - Bhanumati Commentary by *Chakrapani Datta*, Swami Lakshmi RamTrust, Jaipur 1939.

- *Sushruta Samhita* (Three Volumes) - Prof. K.R. Srikantha Murthy, Chaukhamba Orientalia Varanasi.

- *Sushruta Samhita* (*Sootra Sthana*) – Original text & Hindi translation of the *NibandhaSamgraha* Commentary of Shri Dalhanacarya, R.A.V. New Delhi.

- *Yogaratnakara* -Vd. Lakshmipatta Shastri, Chaukhambha Sanskrit Sansthana, Varanasi, Seventh Edition, 1999.

- *Ashtanga Hridayam* with the commentaries, *Sarvangasundara* of *Arundatta* and *Ayurveda Rasayana* of *Hemadri,* editedby *Pandit Hari Sadasiva Sastri Paradakara Bhisagacharya*; Chaukhamba Orientalia, Varanasi, Ninth Edition, 2002.

- *Vachaspatyam (Brhat Sanskrtabhidhanam) Tarka Vacaspati* Shri Taranath Bhattacarya, Vol.1 to 5, Choukhamba Sanskrit Series Office, 1962.

- *Ashtanga Samgraha* - Commentary of Indu, Vol.1 to 3. Central Council for Research in Ayurved and Siddha, New Delhi, 1988.

- *Bhavaprakash Nighantu* - Hindi Commentary by *K. C.Chunekar* Chaukhamba Bharati Academy, Varanasi, Reprit 1999.

- *CharakaSamhita* - *AyurvedaDipika* Commentary of *Chakrapanidutta.* Edited by Vaidya Jadavaji Trikamji Acarya; Chaukhamba Sanskrit Sansthana Varanasi; Fifth Edition, 2001.

- *Charaka Samhita* - Gulabakunwarba Ayurvedic Society, Jamnagar 1949.

- *Charaka Samhita* -Ramkarana Sharma and Bhagwan Dash, Vol.1 to 6.

- *Charaka Samhita - Jalpakalpataru* Commentary Gangadhara Edited by V Katumba Shastri Rashtriya Sanskrit Sansthana, New Delhi, 2002.

- *KashyapaSamhita* -by *VriddhaJivaka*, revised by *Vatsya*, Edited by Pandit Hemaraja Sarma; Chaukhamba Sanskrit Sansthana; Eighth edition, 2002.

- *Madhava Nidana with Madhukosa* commentary of Sri Vijayarakshita and Srikanthadatta. Chaukhambha Sanskrpt Sansthana. Thirtieth Edition, 2000.

- *Sharangadhara Samhita* - Commentaries of *Adhamalla's Dipika* and *Kasirama's Gudhartha Dipika*; Chaukhamba Orientalia, Varanasi, Fourth Edition, 2000.

- *Sushruta Samhita* - Kaviraja Ambikadatta Shastri (Part I & II) Chaukhamba Sanskrit Sansthana, Varanasi Fourteenth Edition, 2001.

- *Sushruta Samhita–Nibandha Samgraha* Commentary of Shri Dalhanacarya, Edited by Jadavaji Trikamji Acarya; Chaukhamba Orientalia Varanasi, Seventh Edition 2002.

REFERENCE BOOKS

- *Ayurvediya Maulika Siddhanta* - Prof. V. J. Thakar, GAU, Jamnagar 1985.

- *Purusha Vicaya* - Prof. V. J. Thakar, GAU, Jamnagar 1985.

- *Ayurvediya Kriya Sharira*, Vd. Ranjeetray Desai, Published by Shri Vaidhyanath Ayurved Bhavan Ltd., Samvat 2056.

- *Sharira Tatwa Darshanam Nama Vatadidosa Vijnanam* – Purushottam Sharma Bhisak "Hirlekar", Amaravati, 1942

DICTIONARIES

- *Shabdakalpadruma* - Raja Radhakanta Devam Chaukhamba Sanskrit Series Office, Varanasi, 1961.

- Sanskrit English Dictionary, Monier Williams. The Clarendon Press, Oxford, 1951.

- Sanskrit Hindi Dictionary - V.S. Apte, 1965.

- *Amarakosha* -Amarsinha, IInd Edition, 1976.

- *Ayurvediya Shabda Kosa* - Venimadhava Joshi and N.H. Joshi, Vol. 1 & 2., Maharashtra Sahitya Sanskriti Mandala, Mumbai, 1968.

- *Nyayakosha* by Mahamahopadhyaya Bhimacharya, Jhalakikara, 3rd edition, published by Bhandarkar Oriental Research Institute, 1928, Pune.